No Margin, No Mission

NO MARGIN, NO MISSION

Health-Care Organizations and the Quest for Ethical Excellence

STEVEN D. PEARSON, M.D., M.Sc.
JAMES E. SABIN, M.D.
EZEKIEL J. EMANUEL, M.D., Ph.D.

With contributions from
TRACEY HYAMS, J.D., M.P.H.
LAUREN RANDEL, M.D.

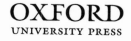

OXFORD
UNIVERSITY PRESS

2003

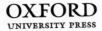

UNIVERSITY PRESS

Oxford   New York
Auckland   Bangkok   Buenos Aires   Cape Town   Chennai
Dar es Salaam   Delhi   Hong Kong   Istanbul   Karachi   Kolkata
Kuala Lumpur   Madrid   Melbourne   Mexico City   Mumbai
Nairobi   São Paulo   Shanghai   Taipei   Tokyo   Toronto

Copyright © 2003 by Oxford University Press, Inc.

Published by Oxford University Press, Inc.
198 Madison Avenue, New York, New York 10016

http://www.oup-usa.org

Oxford is a registered trademark of Oxford University Press

Library of Congress Cataloging-in-Publication Data
No margin, no mission : health-care organizations and the quest for ethical excellence/
Steven D. Pearson, James E. Sabin, Ezekiel J. Emanuel ;
with contributions from Tracey Hyams, Lauren Randel.
p. cm.   Includes bibliographical references and index.
ISBN 0-19-515896-2 (cloth)
1. Managed care plans (Medical care)—Moral and ethical aspects—United States.
2. Health facilities—Moral and ethical aspects.
3. Medical ethics.
I. Pearson, Steven D.
II. Sabin, James E.
III. Emanuel, Ezekiel J., 1957–
RA413.N6 2003   174'.2—dc21   2002041649

9 8 7 6 5 4 3 2 1

Printed in the United States of America
on acid-free paper

To our families

Preface

Our goal in this book is to weave ethical analysis and real-world experience together with a strong, practical, intellectual thread. And, like the golden thread that allowed Theseus to find his way out of the dark, twisting labyrinth of the Minotaur, we hope this book will provide a pathway to valuable lessons for those bold enough to venture into the den of the United States's brand of managed care. If readers emerge refreshed, emboldened, and equipped with new ideas in their own quest for ethical excellence in health care, then this book will have fulfilled its purpose.

But it is reasonable to ask: Why venture in at all? Isn't managed care a failed idea, one encumbered with all the ignominious trappings of capitalist markets run amok? Nations with universal health insurance should find nothing of interest here. Isn't the lesson to be learned from managed care the sad fact that competitive markets place such stress on health-care organizations that ethical excellence is one of the first casualties?

We hope to draw readers toward different conclusions. It is true that the hopes of the last decade for a reborn U.S. health care system lie in disarray. Conflict and stagnation seem the heirs of a once buoyant vision. Yet, even if managed care in the United States is "dead," as some claim, its great challenges—and great opportunities—still face us.

Rising health-care costs still afflict the United States, as they do all other advanced nations. New technologies and aging populations drive the desire for health-care services higher and higher. But as important as health is, it remains only one of many valued social goals. And thus, health-care organizations, both public and private, must cope with the ethical tensions generated by considering costs as well as the quality of health care.

These are the ethical tensions that every advanced health care system faces. No nation seems immune. Norway, Sweden, Canada, Great Britain, the Netherlands: not one of these countries, despite their decades of experience with universal health insurance, has proven invulnerable to the hard choices, tough compromises, and public disappointments of managing care within a budget. Health-care organizations in the United States, responsible for care and its cost, carry many of the same burdens as national health systems and can face the additional challenge of needing to consider individual and organizational profits as part of the delicate ethical balancing act they are asked to perform. Over the past decade, even countries with universal health insurance have sought to graft the entrepreneurial spark and consumer accountability of competitive markets onto the bureaucratic culture of their national health systems.

More and more, health-care organizations and systems are being asked to care for individual patients, keep down costs for all, and manage the tensions between these two goals fairly, all while competing for economic survival in the marketplace. Success in the marketplace thus becomes the primary prerequisite for achieving other goals; hence, the title of this book: "No [profit] Margin, No [health] Mission." The sharp truth behind this oft-repeated phrase presents all nations with a universal ethical and political challenge: How can patients, providers, and the public trust in the legitimacy and fairness of the organizations that provide health care in competitive systems?

We believe that over the past decade the health-care system of the United States, despite its storied ethical deficiencies and singular lapses, has provided a valuable laboratory for seeking answers to this question. Nearly every U.S. health-care organization, in diverse health care markets across the country, has faced the dilemma of how to provide the best health care possible despite resource constraints and market competition. This book presents the results of a two-year national project to make use of this natural laboratory. Named BEST—Best Ethical STrategies for Managed Care—the project was led by our team of investigators at Harvard Medical School, Harvard Pilgrim Health Care, and the National Institutes of Health. Involving the participation of eight large managed care organizations across the country, the goal of the BEST project was to develop an ethical template for exemplary ethical performance and then use this theoretical structure as a foundation from which to study the experience of health-care organizations that have wrestled to design policies and programs that reasonably balance competing values in the marketplace. In this book we explore what the organizations participating in the BEST project told us were some of the toughest decisions in health care today: How can health plans determine what services should be covered as medically necessary in a way that ensures quality care, controls costs, and builds trust with patients and physicians? What are the best strategies for caring for vulnerable populations that can meet their special needs without dramatically increasing costs? How and how much should a health-care organization contribute directly to the community in which it operates?

To answer these and similar questions, we use a pragmatic method that blends ethical analysis with real-world examples. We try to make the ethical dilemmas more accessible to resolution by moving from ethical analysis to field example and back again. The outcome is a rich analysis of the ethical challenges facing health-care organizations, combined with tangible examples of exemplary methods to address these challenges. We hope this book will help health-care leaders, providers, policy makers, and the general public work together to build and sustain exemplary ethical health-care organizations, both in the United States and around the world. Through our book, we invite the reader into the challenging depths of the U.S. experience of health care in competitive markets. Our hope is that the intellectual thread we have fashioned is strong enough to lead one back into the light with a clear understanding of how to develop practical, yet widely applicable, programs of ethical excellence.

The BEST project arose as an idea in conversations among the three of us when we were all working in Boston in the mid 1990s. Later it became a collaborative effort between faculty in the Center for Ethics in Managed Care at Harvard Medical School and Harvard Pilgrim Health Care, and faculty in the Department of Clinical Bioethics at the National Institutes of Health (NIH). Lauren Randel, at the NIH, and Tracey Hyams, in Boston, contributors to this book, were key members of the research team. They both participated in several site visits and worked with us to develop the framework for our ethical analyses. Each also took the lead in writing a chapter in the book (L. Randel, The Care of Vulnerable Populations; T. Hyams, The Confidentiality of Personal Health Information). Their contributions to the BEST project and to this book are truly substantial.

A number of foundations have supported our work. We gratefully acknowledge the generosity of the Henry J. Kaiser Family Foundation, the Seaver Institute, the Nathan Cummings Foundation, and the Robert Wood Johnson Foundation, all of whose financial support was central to the conduct of the project and the writing of this book. Dr. Pearson was also supported as a faculty fellow of the Harvard University Center for Ethics in the Professions during the year when much of the manuscript was written.

We also gratefully acknowledge the central role of the health care organizations that participated fully in the BEST project: Blue Cross Blue Shield of Tennessee, Foundation Health Plan of Florida, Inc., Group Health Cooperative of Puget Sound, Harvard Pilgrim Health Care, Health Net, Holy Cross Health Systems, and the University of Pittsburgh Medical Center Health Plan. These organizations were much more than passive project sites. Each gave us unstinting encouragement, as well as access to leaders and other staff, and helped us, through innumerable conversations and communications, to develop the intellectual structure of this book. This book could not have been written without their openness, honesty, and eagerness to be ethically exemplary organizations.

We also thank many individuals who have offered us criticism and support during the time we have pursued these ideas. Martha Minow, Arthur Applbaum, and the faculty fellows at the Harvard Center for Ethics in the Professions gave valuable feedback on early drafts of several chapters. Steve Shortell offered invaluable advice on how to include ethical considerations in a study of health care organizations. Stefan C. Weiss offered valuable criticism, and many of our primary contacts at the participating BEST organizations also engaged significantly in reviewing and commenting on our work; among these were Bruce Chernoff (Health Net), Jack Gallagher (Holy Cross Health Systems), Rick Miller (Blue Cross Blue Shield of Tennessee), Andrea Voytko (Group Health Cooperative of Puget Sound), Loren Roth (University of Pittsburgh Medical Center Health Plan), and Ralph Fuccillo (Harvard Pilgrim Health Care). Any errors that remain in our book occur despite the best efforts of these individuals to correct our early drafts.

We thank Cynthia Meyers for her unstinting attention to detail in the formatting and final preparation of the manuscript. We wish also to acknowledge the contributions of our many colleagues in the Department of Ambulatory Care and Prevention at Harvard Medical School and Harvard Pilgrim Health Care, and at the Department of Clinical Bioethics at the National Institutes of Health. Despite all the ribbing we took about how any book on exemplary ethical practices in managed care would be notable for its brevity, our colleagues' encouragement, support, and friendship were instrumental in sustaining us through the years it took to bring this work to fruition. Critical *and* supportive, they have been colleagues in the best sense.

Boston, Massachusetts	S.D.P.
Boston, Massachusetts	J.E.S.
Bethesda, Maryland	E.J.E.

Contents

No Margin, No Mission

1

VIRTUE AMONG THE RUINS?

> Health care costs are being treated as if they were largely an economic problem, but they are not. To be solved they will have to be treated as an ethical problem.
>
> Lester Thurow*

There is an urgency to this book, an urgency born of concern and hope. The concern is easy to understand. The American health-care system is in a state of crisis. Basic health coverage remains out of reach to millions of citizens, while the cost of care for the insured population has resumed a rapid rate of increase that promises to price ever more employers and individuals out of the health-care insurance market. Administrative costs remain the highest in the world. Despite spending more on health care than any other nation in the world, the U.S. health-care system is plagued by medical errors and failures to provide proven clinical "best practices,"—the screening tests, preventive care, and medical treatments known to be most effective. Broad efforts to reform the system have met with public suspicion and skepticism, a reaction reinforced by the failure of the Clinton health-care initiative of the 1990s. Even limited reform efforts often sink into a quagmire of selfishness and distrust. Powerful interests, including managed care insurers, pharmaceutical corporations, and hospitals and physicians, line up to combat each other or to fend off regulatory efforts sponsored by citizens' groups or the government. We have power without vision, conflict without progress. The system is stuck.

Of course, it wasn't supposed to be this way. Once there was a powerful idea for the basis of a better U.S. health-care system. The experience of large, prepaid

*Thurow, L. D. Learning to say "no." *New England Journal of Medicine* 1987; 311 (24): 1569–1572.

group practices, such as Kaiser Permanente, Group Health Cooperative of Puget Sound, and Harvard Community Health Plan, had shown that excellent health care, with an emphasis on prevention and primary care, could be provided by integrated delivery systems at a significant cost savings compared with traditional fee-for-service practice. Visionaries like Paul Ellwood foresaw the extension of the HMO (health maintenance organization) model bringing benefits to the entire U.S. population, with lower health-care costs enabling our society to pursue seriously the elusive goal of universal insurance coverage. In the minds of many, managed care would eventually become the midwife to a national health system promising universal access, delivering high-quality care, and founded upon values of community health and social justice.

Today the United States seems permanently estranged from this vision. But progress is more likely to come from stubborn optimism and hard work than from despair and resignation. If the goal is to advance the quality of health care for all members of society, we must find examples and insights to guide us toward that end. But where will we find these examples? Many have touted as models the industrialized nations that have decades of experience with national health insurance. The United Kingdom, Sweden, Canada, Germany, and others have provided valuable examples of the ethical and political courage that the United States will have to muster if it is to achieve universal health insurance. The various specific structures that these nations have developed to finance and administer their health-care systems can also serve as important models that could be adapted for use in the United States. Many American ethicists and policy makers have long looked abroad with admiration and hope.

The usefulness of other nations' experiences has been limited, however, by persistent fears that it would be difficult or impossible to graft successfully other health-care models onto the American cultural and political foundation. Critics find it easy to point out that the health-care systems of other nations have had plenty of their own problems, including difficulty maintaining professional and public satisfaction with the quality of care (Blendon et al., 1990). Even more fundamental, according to this line of thinking, is the belief that, without a major social catastrophe, the United States is simply too individualistic, or too capitalistic, or too influenced by physicians, or too politically inert, to accept a radically redesigned health care system based on a social ethic of communitarian concern (Emanuel, 1991; Fuchs, 1998). The debacle of the Clinton health care proposal strongly reinforced this notion, and thus the dominant health-care policy approach in the United States has become one of nearly unquestioned incrementalism.

But an atmosphere of incrementalism need not spell the death of high ideals nor forestall important progress. We can improve the present system while preparing for the future. Managed care, as traditionally conceived, may indeed be "dead," as some critics have claimed (Robinson, 2001). Consumers, bewitched by the notion that choice of physician is paramount and enticed by pharmaceutical companies to satisfy the national taste for the newest and "best" in modern treatment and technology, have rejected most of the traditional means used by insurers to seek rationalization and cost-control in health care. Perhaps the future holds only more of this brand of consumerism, with purchasers and insurers continuing to disengage and managed care organizations ultimately reduced to crafting the actuarial nuances of deductibles and tiered co-payments. Other analysts hold out the hope that the U.S. health-care system is on a slow march to an ultimate destination of some kind of national health program, one in which universal insurance and federal control will end the fragmented market-oriented approach and revolutionize the assumptions of what managed care should be.

One thing, however, is certain. Whatever health-care system lies in the future for the United States, it will still have to cope with ethical tensions generated by considering costs and access as well as the quality of care. Priorities will need to be set; hard choices and the inevitable disappointment of some will prove inescapable. This is the central ethical tension that every advanced health-care system faces. And today, despite the managed care malaise in this country, we have before us in the current health-care system of the United States a valuable laboratory for learning about ethical and clinical excellence. Nearly every U.S. health-care organization has faced in the past decade the dilemma of how to provide the best health care possible within resource constraints while facing stiff market competition. Of failure, moral cowardice, and outright greed, the stories have been plentiful (Anders, 1996). Certainly, no single health-care organization is perfect; many, however, can point with pride to some policies, structures, or processes, often created anew after the cleansing fire of a previous public disaster, that embody exemplary ethical features. These exemplary practices come with lessons learned and insights gained from which all can benefit. Health-care organizations, physicians, patients, legislators, the press—all want to see health care managed well today, with a clear pathway to continued improvement. The future of the U.S. health-care system will depend on the maturity of its vision of how to manage the tension between caring and cost. The same can be said of the challenge facing other developed countries. Thus, the time is ripe for analyzing the ethical lessons of organizations facing the tough choices and tight budgets of the present U.S. health-care system. Examining closely the lessons learned during this period should help provide a guide to sustaining ethical excellence in all health-care systems molded by the influence of competitive markets.

MANAGED CARE, AMERICAN STYLE

Although prepaid health care plans had been growing slowly over the decades since Kaiser and Group Health Cooperative pioneered the concept, the real push toward managed care came during the late 1980s when large employers and the federal government faced the sticker shock of rising health-care costs. The major purchasers of health-care insurance recognized the need to control costs and set health-care priorities, but the United States was burdened by a culture and history that idealized individual choice while denying the reality of resource limits. Following the failure of the Clinton health-care proposal in the 1990s, and with scant political leadership willing to lead a national debate on the tough choices necessary in health-care funding, purchasers and policy makers followed the well-beaten path back to a different solution: the market. *Managed competition*, a system of market competition among large insurance companies to deliver prepaid health care, became the default U.S. health-care policy. Competition, it was hoped, would retain choice as a key value underlying the health-care system. Competition would ensure efficiency while keeping insurers and providers responsive to their customers; lower costs and better primary care, prevention, and coordination would be among its beneficial by-products. It seemed simple: the market would maximize value, and everyone would be satisfied with the result.

High hopes can be rudely disappointed. Even the most doubtful of critics, however, were unlikely to have foreseen the degree of public loathing for which managed care has become the poster child. As managed care was extended beyond the self-selected minority of patients in the older HMOs to ever-larger segments of the working public, an anti–managed-care backlash rose to contest it. It did not help that the new HMOs were often operated by large, for-profit companies with no tradition of commitment to preventive care, whose cost-control leverage over loose provider networks was limited to heavy-handed utilization management techniques. "1-800-JUST SAY NO" jokes abounded; lampooning cartoons and negative media portrayals, as in the movies *As Good As it Gets* and *John Q*, became commonplace. Regulators and state legislative representatives across the country soon found that managed care was a popular, convenient, and politically expedient target. Both Democrats and Republicans ultimately endorsed a patients' bill of rights as protection against managed care (Goldstein and Eilperin, 1998; Grunwald, 1999). And the lawyers who successfully sued the tobacco companies and are currently pursuing gun manufacturers turned their sights toward major health plans (Segal and Goldstein, 1999).

What does the U.S. public see when it looks at managed care? Many see large, insensitive corporations more interested in profits than in patients' health (Kaiser Family Foundation, 1997). The public believes that health-care executives reap fat bonus packages while needed health-care services are denied to save money and boost stock prices, that access is blocked to specialists and high-technology services, that financial incentives provide physicians a "fee for no service," and that patient confidentiality may be violated to discover and target high-cost users (Annas, 1998).

Faced with the deepening distrust of the public, how have managed care organizations responded? Many have shared a sense of dismay, mixed with resignation, at being caught, as they see it, between a rock and a hard place. Purchasers demand lower costs, rarely using quality as the basis for their purchasing decisions. The public resents any restraints on health care. Since neither public officials nor purchasers are willing to admit that health-care resources are limited and that tough choices must be made, managed care companies have found it nearly impossible to unmask these realities themselves in the context of market competition. After all, what would the fate be of the health plan that courageously ventured to be the first in its market to promote how effectively it rations health care?

And so, managed care organizations, feeling misunderstood by the public and undeservedly maligned by a biased press, can only share in private their sense of disillusion and suffering for what they view as a noble cause. In public, they have tried just about everything to win the battle of perceptions. A number of health plans have adopted public relations campaigns that highlight their accountability and their commitment to high-quality medical care (Pear, 1997). They cite data showing that managed care enrollees have as high, if not higher, satisfaction rates as fee-for-service patients; and they point to higher immunization rates and studies demonstrating that managed care is equivalent to, if not superior to, fee-for-service medicine on a variety of quality measures (Aetna U.S. Healthcare, 1999; National Committee for Quality Assurance, 2001). They also argue that, unlike the physicians and hospitals in the old fee-for-service system, managed care organizations are being held accountable for the quality of their outcomes through a myriad of formal and explicit "report cards." But all of these efforts seem to have fallen on deaf ears. What managed care is selling, the public does not seem to be buying.

The managed care industry's response clearly has not connected with the public. The result has been a true breakdown in trust between the American public and its health care system. Without trust, little accommodation can be given to different perspectives, and very few opportunities for mutual listening and learning can succeed. Unfortunately, there are few examples of effective means of public participation and common deliberation within health-care institutions: The public is essentially on the outside looking in, and too often the most effective way to communicate seems to be to lob bricks over the high wall. Legal remedies appear to be the only avenue for change. But change seems less likely than ever as purchasers, managed care organizations, and the public, facing each other uncomprehendingly, dig in their heels. It is now difficult to sense any chance of progress toward a broader societal consensus about the U.S. health-care system. Critical questions about health care lie before the nation: cost, access, quality, justice. In an atmosphere of heat without light, of politicization without political leadership, the risk is that the current conflict over managed care will continue to lead only to stagnation.

A NEW APPROACH

Given the other reasons favoring incrementalism in U.S. health-care policy, the irreconcilable conflicts brought into focus by managed care cast a pall over the entire health-care system. But the premise of this book is that the public debate over managed care can be transformed by reframing political and clinical conflicts as examples of ethical tension or as conflicts of values arising from the attempt to use disparate organizations, operating under the strictures of market competition, to graft together a patient- and population-centered approach to health care. As we will show, seemingly intractable problems, arising in areas as diverse as benefit and medical necessity determinations, the care of vulnerable populations, confidentiality, and consumer voice in health-care decisions, can be disentangled and approached more constructively when viewed as the ethical dilemmas they really are.

Ethics, in our view, offers a useful lens through which to evaluate conflicts in the U.S. system of managed care, and it also provides a specific model for collaborative, reflective change. But what kind of ethics are we talking about—normative? descriptive? meta-ethics? There are ethical approaches, well known in health care, that are dominated by a particular philosophical principle. For example, libertarian market ethics posits that the ethics of individual freedom, along with its corollary of the free exercise of capitalist markets, together provide the framework for justifying unhindered competition as the answer to health-care woes (Englehardt, 1996; Epstein, 1998). There are ethics approaches that are framed in terms of a simple dichotomy of ideologies: medicine vs. business (Relman, 1992; Kassirer, 1995). Other ethics methods have also sought to focus their analyses within simplifying categories, such as conflict of interest, consent, or choice (Anderlik, 2001).

The ethics approach adopted in this book is quite different. It is an applied ethics whose philosophic method could best be labeled pragmatic (Wolf, 1994; McGee, 1999). The characteristic idea of philosophical pragmatism is that efficacy in practical application provides a standard for the determination of truth in the case of statements, rightness in the case of actions, and value in the case of appraisals (Fins et al., 1998). The pragmatic ethical tradition, which traces its roots to the American philosophers Charles Sanders Peirce, William James, and John Dewey, focuses on problems and promotes inquiry and deliberation, with judgments rigorously linked to revision on the basis of further experience and learning. Inclusive of claims and concerns from both consequentialist and deontological perspectives, pragmatic ethics is underpinned by a distinctly democratic vision and, at its best, results in the "creative melding of insights from various sources to address social problems" (Anderlik, 2001, p. 46).

Physicians, health care executives, and policy experts in the United States may be able to recognize this methodology as an extension of what they have witnessed as the most routine form of bioethics, the hospital *ethics consult*. Part of the bioethics tradition is case consultation—attempting to advise in particular patient-care situations where there are value conflicts and a pressing need for a solution that is simultaneously practical and ethically justifiable. The pragmatic approach we take in this book is in many ways deeply rooted in this tradition of applied bioethics, where synergy is constantly sought between case-based experience and ethical theory. Another aspect of the bioethics tradition is the recognition that despite disagreement about abstract ethical theories, there can be what is called an *overlapping consensus* on particular values and the ethical resolution of actual cases. Throughout this book we have mirrored this pragmatic approach, intentionally moving back and forth between ethical values and empirical realities. This approach could also be called *evidence-based ethical analysis*, for we have not sought to magically derive *ought* from *is*, but rather, we have found the ethical dilemmas much more accessible to discussion, insight, and possible solution by moving from consideration of pure ethical values to field example and back again.

This book is, therefore, an experiment in pragmatic ethics as a method of analysis and change in health care. Such a method must compete in the marketplace of ideas not only with other approaches to ethics but with quite different approaches to "fixing" health care, including those that are regulatory (pass a patients' bill of rights), economic (create new financing systems or universal insurance), political (put the power in some other hands), or managerial (adopt new organizational structures). Our method of using pragmatic ethics as a lens with which to examine organizational dilemmas in the health-care system will not suit everyone. Some may think our approach shares the drawbacks that have been associated with ethics in general as a method of analysis and as a tool for health policy change. For example, some believe that ethics of any stripe may be ill suited for the role of organizational analysis. Bioethics has clearly served well as a tool for analyzing the narrow conflicts of individual doctor–patient relationships. But perhaps it is not well suited to the task of tackling issues in the broader arena of organizations, where economics and health policy rule the day. Linked to this concern is the belief that ethics can be too vague, too relativistic, to achieve any concrete progress. Why abandon hard-headed tactics like legislative regulation and enforcement to embrace a more reflective method that has no teeth?

A different criticism of the pragmatic ethics methodology we have used is that it comes from inside the system; it may be co-opted by exposure to the rough and tumble of market realities, and thus emerge too sympathetic to the status quo. Pragmatic philosophy has always been vulnerable to concerns that its standards for judgment are too instrumental, ultimately yielding to expediency. The controversies in the U.S. health-care system can only heighten the concern that larger ethical goals will be sacrificed to a superficial satisfaction with "what works now." According to an extreme version of this view, the U.S. health-care system is fatally flawed and so inherently unethical that any kind of pragmatic ethical analysis smacks of accommodation. The U.S. system ignores universal access, siphons health-care resources into the pockets of investors and executives, and strips away patient–physician autonomy as it subverts the ethical value of caring for the individual. There is no reason to bargain with this devil; ethics is useful only insofar as it can be used to condemn the U.S. managed care experiment. Trying to use ethics to pretty it up piecemeal would be like improving the efficiency of the engines on the Titanic.

We reject these arguments and believe that looking at the current conflict through the lens of pragmatic, evidence-based ethics alters the strategies for solving the current health care crisis and offers several distinct advantages in guiding the United States and other developed health-care systems toward a better future. First, ethical analysis of organizations and systems in health care can help achieve the same goals that effective bioethics consultation can attain in other areas: clarification of terms; search for input from multiple perspectives; delineation of values; explicit prioritization of values; and exploration of potential new solutions. Ethics can help decision makers reach a reflective equilibrium rarely otherwise achieved in the fast-paced organizational life that is one of the by-products of market competition. In addition, pragmatic ethics as a health-policy tool need not exclude other options and, in fact, by increasing dialogue, ethics may help build coalitions and potentiate the effectiveness of other avenues for social pressure and change. We believe that ethics is tough enough to be the central tool of effective change.

To those who would argue that the U.S. managed care system is inherently unethical, we hope to demonstrate in this book that there are nuggets of gold to be found in the attitudes and approaches of some managed care organizations. Through these lessons, even if scattered and incomplete, ethics can help frame a positive track toward the future. Part of this positive framing ability comes from the fact that an ethics approach, when grounded in real-world experience, must acknowledge that ethical tensions are inherent in all health-care systems and that the shift to managed care in the United States has highlighted many of these tensions. Pragmatic ethics, instead of offering up broad utopian vistas, helps build a consensus that there is, in fact, nowhere to hide from tough choices. There is no way a modern health-care system can avoid the dilemmas posed by caring and cost or by providing the best possible care to individuals within the constraints of the resources society is willing to devote to health care. Indeed, these conflicts are surfacing in all Western countries from Canada and Germany to Norway and Sweden. By acknowledging ethical tensions born out of value conflicts, the ethics lens serves to force various stakeholders to accept the validity of the perspectives and values of others. An explicit pragmatic ethics approach encourages respect for others' opinions. And where there is respect, there is an opportunity for listening, learning, and positive change.

Perhaps most importantly, in a health-care world of tough situations and hard choices, pragmatic ethics can provide a model for a systematic decision-making process, a process that can be perceived by all stakeholders to be legitimate (Daniels and Sabin, 2002). In representative democracies the distance between the public and political decision makers gives rise to the call for open meetings, formal rules of procedure, and even decision-making methods that purport to be objective (Gutmann and Thompson, 1996). In the U.S. health-care system, for example, even if the profit motive were not a concern, there is ample reason for the public to seek a similar level of transparency and objectivity to important health care decisions. For if Americans do not know their physicians due to the rise of group practices, if their health plans are switched from year to year by employers seeking lower prices, and if their increased residential mobility leads to fractured health-care relationships, then Americans will not know, or trust, the values of the decision makers who control their health care. And so it is true, to a greater or lesser degree, among all developed nations, that not having personal interaction to build trust in decision makers, the public turns to a search for a decision-making *process* in which it can trust.

What are the core elements of a trustworthy process? The public looks foremost for two things: (*1*) a chance to have its voice heard; and (*2*) observable rules by which it can feel that it understands how decisions are reached. The pragmatic ethical lens is best understood as a method of inquiry and decision making that has these core building blocks of legitimacy. This is so because the style of inquiry at the heart of pragmatic ethics involves having a "positive regard for the experience, intelligence, and humanity of others" (Anderlik, 2001, p. 56). It allows us to examine the conflicts of values among competing interests, each of which represents a reasonable, justifiable position. And even when there are fundamentally irreconcilable value conflicts, a pragmatic approach offers a way to find common ground, implement values practically, and achieve a level of legitimacy necessary to move forward in improving health-care systems. Pragmatic ethics certainly has its risks and disadvantages. But the adoption of universal moral respect and reciprocity and the cultivation of the ability to take the standpoint of the other are the foundation upon which democratic deliberation can be realized.

"NO MISSION, NO MARGIN" AND THE ETHICAL STRESS TEST OF MANAGED CARE

When training as a student in medical school, one often learns clinical "pearls"—bite-sized pieces of condensed wisdom meant to help novices synthesize data in complex clinical situations and figure out what to do. Classics such as "If you think of it, do it," (when considering a spinal tap to evaluate a patient with a headache) and "Never let the sun go down on a small bowel obstruction," (when deciding whether surgery is needed immediately for a patient with abdominal pain) are not just created for the snappy dialogue on *E.R.* but have, in fact, long figured in the education of physicians, much to the chagrin of theorists of evidence-based clinical thinking.

Complex, difficult choices; easy, straightforward answers. Given the former, the human need for the latter seems universal. Thus it is that when faced with time and resource pressures in market-based health care, it is all too easy to collapse personal, and even organizational, reflection into similar snippets of wisdom to manage difficult choices. One of the favorites we heard frequently during the BEST project was "No margin, no mission." In other words, if you don't make a profit, you can't hope to pursue whatever beneficial mission you have in mind for the organization. So, be tough, make the hard choice, hope for tomorrow. This axiom seemed to be on the lips of leaders at many of the proud, old-guard HMOs, organizations born in idealism and rooted in a culture of community health and progress. But the same words were commonplace at for-profit HMOs across the country as well. In the tight and turbulent health-care markets of the mid-to-late 1990s, organizations across the spectrum of the managed care system faced economic life-or-death struggles that put tremendous stress on the traditional ethical balances that had been struck in the past: Short-term profit vs. commitment to serve vulnerable populations; confidentiality of member information vs. requests from influential consultants and brokers for more information; preventive health care vs. purchasers' requests for stripped-out benefit packages. Whatever the organizational positions had been on these tensions in the past were now old news. With survival often at stake, all the previous assumptions were up for grabs.

"No margin, no mission." It is easy to imagine how many ethically complex, important business decisions in managed health care could be quickly made in deference to a simple interpretation of this seemingly benign axiom. And yet, we believe that most health care organizations, whether in times of dire economic stress or in those of relative prosperity, really do want to be sensitive to the ethical tensions inherent in what they must do to balance care and cost in a competitive market. Organizations we met with seemed hungry for even the most critical feedback. They wanted a road map for change, and they wanted tested methods to improve their attention to ethical values. It is our ultimate hope that through the process of defining ethical values in conflict and then highlighting innovative and effective organizational strategies to manage that conflict, we will be able to spark internal ethical reflection across many different kinds of health-care organizations.

The goal of this book, therefore, is to provide a path for collaborative change. To achieve this end, we have included insights and examples that should appeal to multiple audiences. Health plan Chief Executive Officers and medical directors, hospital executives, and leaders of provider groups that have risk-bearing contracts—all may find examples of exemplary practices they can voluntarily adapt and implement. Health-care organizations may come to understand their own problems more clearly as value conflicts and adapt and develop exemplary practices to manage their ethical tensions. Furthermore, these organizations may come to see the role of openness and inclusive decision making in regaining public trust. Regulators at the state and federal level, or in agencies such as the Joint Commission on Accreditation of Healthcare Organizations (JCAHO) or the National Committee for Quality Assurance (NCQA), may look to the analyses and examples in this book in devising creative new legislative and accreditation standards. Regulators and legislators may move away from mandates of specific services and bills of rights to encourage more innovative ethical strategies such as public education and open decision making.

Physicians and other health-care professionals, seeking an understanding of the current conflicts in managed care and of the potential role they can play in improving the ethical quality of care for their patients, will also find much in this book to guide them.

And finally, consumer advocates, legislators, and the media may use the analyses and exemplary practices described in this book to help frame a positive direction in which to influence the health-care system. Consumers may change their demands from the right to sue to a broader goal: getting health care organizations to adopt exemplary ethical practices. Members of the public may come to appreciate the complexity of the allocation decisions society faces and be motivated to educate themselves and participate in decision making. Ultimately, through improved dialogue and understanding, our hope is that it will be possible for the United States and other societies to come to terms with the larger ethical issues facing all health-care systems. In this book, step by step, organization by organization, we may find insights into how, with limited resources, we can yet care for all of us with justice and compassion.

2

EVIDENCE-BASED ETHICS AND
THE BEST PROJECT

The BEST project and its accompanying ethical analysis were conceived of and directed by a collaborative research team from Harvard Medical School, Harvard Pilgrim Health Care, and the National Institutes of Health. Our team included individuals with training and experience in philosophy, law, public health, health services research, and health-care management. Multidisciplinary in background, the team was distinguished by the fact that all but one member was a physician still active in part-time clinical practice. It is well known that physicians and physician-ethicists may bring their own strongly forged clinical culture to the table in any ethical forum. With an internist, an oncologist, and two psychiatrists participating, we were endowed with a full measure of clinical cultures from the quite different worlds of primary care, specialty care, and mental health. In addition to varying clinical cultures, the mix of physician specialties gave us a broad range of exposures to the managed care experience of practicing physicians in the United States. Our personal experiences included, among others, coming face to face with closed formularies, onerous 1-800 utilization-approval phone numbers, rapid shifts in approved provider lists for specialty referral, and disputes over funding experimental treatment protocols. One of us even had his part-time clinical position eliminated in a wave of cost cutting during the course of the BEST project.

These negative experiences notwithstanding, two of us (Pearson and Sabin) have carried out most of our clinical and research work within what used to be known

13

as a managed care setting. We had both worked in the organization that had a long life as Harvard Community Health Plan and eventually became Harvard Pilgrim Health Care. Our personal experience in managed care included participation in the early years of nonprofit HMOs when the ideal of community health and solidarity was a moving force. We felt the electricity of the early charismatic, visionary leaders whose bedrock principles of patient care and public health were unshakeable.

Being part of a staff-model HMO had also given us the chance to practice in a purely salaried, integrated, multispecialty group practice, driven by professional culture and strong peer relationships. Formal measures of the quality of care were as high, if not higher, than anywhere else in the country. As members of this large prepaid group practice we had also witnessed, and hope we did not contribute to, the Achilles heel of staff-model HMOs: a clinic structure and mentality that felt less personal and more bureaucratic to some patients when compared to smaller, more independent medical groups. Through it all, we had been colleagues of the HMO's leadership—men and women seeking to bring prevention and high-quality care to a defined population while nurturing an organizational mission that explicitly included teaching and research. Their vision of a better health-care system was compelling.

It should be noted that we witnessed this entire heritage come under tremendous pressure in the years leading up to the initiation of the BEST project. The market forces that led to the evolution of Harvard Community Health Plan into Harvard Pilgrim Health Care and then ultimately threatened Harvard Pilgrim Health Care's very existence made a seamless transmission of culture over the years impossible. The financial and ethical stress test of the late 1990s forced ever harder choices on HMOs across the nation. Harvard Pilgrim Health Care was no exception, and we were there to witness the struggle for its soul.

The close association of some of the authors with Harvard Pilgrim Health Care raises an additional point. Although originally from many regions of the United States and despite being engaged with research partners across the country and around the world, most members of the research team have spent their professional lives largely in Massachusetts. Massachusetts, and New England, generally, is known as the home of many (some would say too many) academic medical institutions, whose commitment to their own brand of clinical care, research, and education has colored the medical and health-care culture of the entire region. In part due to the influence of these academic health centers, Massachusetts has had only the most peripheral experience with for-profit hospitals and insurers. Instead, prestigious academic hospitals such as the Brigham and Women's Hospital and Massachusetts General Hospital dominate the hospital scene, while employers and other health-care purchasers can choose from nationally respected not-for-profit insurers, including Harvard Pilgrim Health Care, Tufts Health Plan, Blue Cross Blue Shield of Massachusetts, and Fallon Community Health Plan. New England has not widely experimented with the insurance model of large-scale delegation and shared risk that sent many physician groups into death spirals in California and the West. Nor has New England ever experienced the kind of rapid influx seen in parts of the South and Midwest of transient for-profit insurers who move rapidly into a market by underpricing their product for a short time, scoop up as many enrollees and providers as possible, and then sell out to other firms for a quick profit. Home to relatively stable provider networks and not-for-profit insurers, endowed with a purchaser group largely composed of mid-to-large employers providing stable employment and rich benefit packages, and nourished by health-care premiums higher than anywhere else in the country, New England never saw the worst of the nation's managed care experience.

The authors are thus aware that it is easy to be sanguine when reflecting on the U.S. health-care system from the relative comfort of New England. Perhaps our optimism that dialogue within an ethical process can lead to change is given strength by our exposure to the individuals, organizations, and the health-care market we have known best. It would be a mistake, however, to think that we have not considered this possibility from the inception of our work. We set out at the beginning of the BEST project to inject our experience and insights with fresh perspectives from as broad a sampling of health-care settings and institutions as practical. And so we began in 1995 by inviting a broad spectrum of health-care organizations from across the country to participate as partners in this project. Our goal was not to create a representative sample of health plans but, rather, to seek a mixture of health plans and provider groups, with very different organizational histories, structures, and ideas, in order to create as broad a palette as possible from which to illustrate lessons about the ethical challenges of organizations in managed care.

Responding positively to our invitation were organizations large and small, including leading national for-profit insurers, old-guard, not-for-profit group- and staff-model HMOs, two religiously based provider organizations, and a state-based Blue Cross Blue Shield health plan (see Table 2–1). This group met our goal of diversity in geographical location, tax status, organizational structure, and affiliation. Our original list of invitees included some organizations that did not ultimately participate fully in the project. Even the varied stories of what led certain organizations to decline to join or to drop out of the project reflected what was going on in the U.S. health-care system and helped inform our understanding of the challenges facing many organizations.

Prudential Health Care, for example, was an enthusiastic participant at our first meeting, sharing its hard-won experience in the area of medical necessity determination for experimental treatments of life-threatening illnesses. But Prudential was soon purchased by Aetna, and its unique leadership and organizational culture quickly dissipated in the merger. And Aetna itself, represented early in the BEST project by an enthusiastic senior medical director, ultimately declined to participate, upon the advice of its legal department, which pulled the plug only two days before our scheduled site visit to corporate headquarters.

Table 2–1. Participating organizations in the BEST ("Best Ethical STrategies") Project

	PRIMARY GEOGRAPHIC TERRITORY	APPROXIMATE NUMBER OF ENROLLEES AT BEGINNING OF PROJECT	TAX STATUS
Blue Cross Blue Shield of Tennessee	Tennessee	1,1,500,000	Nonprofit
Foundation Health Plan of Florida	Florida	165,000	For-profit
Group Health Cooperative of Puget Sound	Washington State	600,000	Nonprofit
Harvard Pilgrim Health Care	Massachusetts	1,000,000	Nonprofit
University of Pittsburgh Medical Center Health Plan	Pennsylvania	100,000	Nonprofit
Health Net	California	2,500,000	For-profit
Holy Cross Health System	California and Indiana	Not Applicable	Nonprofit

What was the attraction for organizations to participate in BEST? In a time-pressured and outcome-oriented business, why did most of the organizations we contacted agree to spend their time and effort on this project? We did not try to sell them on the merits of the academic patina that might attend affiliation with the project and its published results. What we offered health-care leaders instead was a quick insight into their own organization and a sharing of exemplary achievements by other organizations in areas of ethical controversy. We argued that by participating in BEST, each organization could learn better how to build and sustain one of its most important strategic assets: public trust. This argument found willing ears.

But why wouldn't health-care organizations be able to do this for themselves? At the very least, one might assume they could learn all they needed to from others through the many managed care conferences or by just by looking around at their competitors. The eagerness with which most of our invited organizations responded confirmed our belief that the pressures of the current marketplace can prevent even the most conscientious organizations from devoting time and resources to the reflective process essential to ethical consideration. The pace of change in the health-care market over the past decade has been dizzying. Corporate strategies across the country have undergone seismic shifts since the mid-1990s, in rapid succession from an early phase of growth at any cost to a market-compelled retrenchment and return to actuarial austerity. This rapid shift of focus and strategy happened during the same time that nearly all organizations in health care were also furiously positioning themselves to be at the forefront of those who would capitalize on the Internet and the subsequent "e-health" movement. And change has not been limited to corporate goals and strategies; even the faces seem to change every couple of months. It has been common over the past decade to return to a health-care organization after a 12-month interval to find that all the senior executives have been replaced. Where is the organizational memory necessary for learning? What employee or executive wants to risk his or her job during tough times by engaging in something as superfluous as "ethics"?

One of the stories we heard during the project captured this sense of intense organizational focus that made ethical reflection difficult. The story came from a senior medical leader who, in describing his organization's current climate, recounted the widely repeated dictum of the current CEO, who had quickly removed several top officers from the company: "We have too many people paying attention to the 'interesting many.' We need to focus on the 'vital few.'" To organizations operating under such conditions, the BEST project offered a relatively painless way to learn about themselves and from others. Insight is often dearly bought in the market, and the BEST project, promising to focus on problems, emphasize lessons of success, and point toward the future, found a ready audience.

The project followed a deliberate sequence of operational steps. First, after establishing our working group of health-care organizations, we held a meeting of senior representatives to discuss their view of the ethical dilemmas facing their organizations. Although the name of the project was "Best Ethical STrategies," we were careful not to frame the opening conversations in terms of ethics. *Ethics* has many different connotations and meanings, some of which we felt would create too narrow a window into the most important dilemmas faced by health-care organizations in competitive markets. We opted instead to ask open-ended questions, hoping to build a taxonomy of ethical issues out of the real problems faced by the executives and senior physicians of these organizations. "Tell us about the problems that keep you up at night." "What kinds of problems does your organization face that will still be a challenge in the future, no matter what legislation or regulation comes along?" "Where did your organization stumble the worst in terms of its trust in the eyes of physicians or patients, and what did you learn from the experience?" These were some of the questions we asked in order to stimulate the thought and conversation of our participants. Following an initial series of two face-to-face meetings in which these questions were explored in depth, the research team began an iterative process with the participating organizations that ultimately led to a classification of the problems and examples raised into a total of seven specific ethical domains (see Table 2–2).

As we moved formally from the framework of problems identified by the health care leaders to a more structured description of overarching ethical domains, we sought to make clear that there were competing ethical *values* in each domain that lay behind the actual problems faced by organizations, often leading to the gut-wrenching feeling described by our participants. Most of the ethical domains we identified are widely recognized and easily understood; some, such as confidentiality and end-of-life care, arise directly from corresponding ethical issues in in-

Table 2–2. Representative organizational problems identified by medical leaders and subsequent ethical domains created for analysis in the BEST project

ORGANIZATIONAL PROBLEMS	ETHICAL DOMAINS
Negative publicity over integration of mental health records within an electronic medical record available to all clinicians	Confidentiality
Increasing demands for medical data from self-insured purchasers and their consultants	
New Health Insurance Portability and Accountability Act (HIPAA) rules and regulations	
Several years of severe operational deficits straining traditional allocation of resources to community benefits	Community Benefits
Increasing state scrutiny of community benefits as justification for nonprofit status	
Pressures from internal executives and boards of directors to demonstrate value for investment in community benefits	
Increasing deficits from Medicare and Medicaid lines of business	Vulnerable Populations
Difficulty designing translation services and other delivery system services for patients from so many cultural backgrounds	
State governmental and regulatory pressures to serve Medicaid patients	
Negative publicity and legal exposure from controversial coverage denials	Medical Necessity, Coverage Decisions, and Medical Policy
Difficulty of linking technology assessment with benefits policy	
Constant tension between rules of coverage and individual cases that may justify benefit exceptions	
Variation in coverage for palliative care and nursing services leading to misunderstandings with patients and families	End-of-Life Care
Difficulty of establishing comprehensive end-of-life care programs across diffuse and varied network of providers	

(continued)

Table 2–2. (*continued*)

ORGANIZATIONAL PROBLEMS	ETHICAL DOMAINS
Efforts to develop specific principles to guide organizational decision making without much impact	Organizational Ethics
Ethics viewed as outside the concern of core business functions	
Ethics groups becoming mouthpieces for discontented, angry, internal constituencies	
Difficulty in finding consumers interested and willing to participate on organizational committees	Consumer Empowerment
Disclosing coverage decision rationales raising fear that consumers and physicians will "game" the system	
Questions of how to invite consumer input without creating unrealistic expectations	

dividual doctor–patient relationships and thus seem relatively straightforward. Other domains are less well-defined constructs that emerged slowly from our continued interactions with the organizations. For instance, the domain of medical necessity, coverage decisions, and medical policy began initially as a focus on the problem of adopting new technologies, then grew to include benefit adjudication, and after that, benefit design. Ultimately, after visiting several health plans, an even broader conception emerged, as we came to see that these areas of concern exist deeply intertwined within the overall organizational approach to medical policy.

All the domains have distinctively *organizational* perspectives that lead ethical analysis beyond the usual academic boundaries that are well mapped out for the ethics of individual doctors and patients. New views on traditional ethical duties and responsibilities caused by the roles of organizations are part of what has triggered the debates and controversies in managed care. We found it useful to delineate the contribution of the organizational perspective within each of the domains and trace the evolution of new views from the traditional focus of bioethics on the individual patient–doctor relationship. Our analysis is shown in Table 2–3. As can be seen, in many of the domains, the role of the organization does not simply augment or facilitate at a distance the role of the individual physician; rather, the organization figuratively steps right into the middle of the doctor–patient relationship, with the potential of disrupting or even usurping the prerogatives previously assigned in splendid isolation to the doctor–patient dyad. It is easy to see

Table 2–3. Domains of ethical tension in health care

DOMAIN	TRADITIONAL FOCUS	NEW VIEW
Confidentiality	A physician protects patient confidences, balanced only by issues of public health and explicit danger to others.	An organization seeks to guard privacy while using clinical information for utilization review, quality improvement, and research.
Community Benefits	A physician provides free care for a needy individual patient.	An organization establishes policies and systems to provide free care and/or other benefits to the community.
Vulnerable Populations	A physician tailors care for a patient with special needs.	An organization accommodates the needs of vulnerable consumers and patients through special policies and systems.
Medical Necessity and Appropriateness	A physician and patient decide when a specific service is in the patient's best interest.	An organization evaluates new interventions for cost-effectiveness and marginal benefit. An organization holds the final say in what will be paid for in the care of the individual patient.
End-of-Life Care	A physician and patient seek to maximize autonomy and quality of life in a series of discrete clinical decisions.	An organization seeks improvement in coordination of end-of-life care services (e.g. timely hospice referral, completed advance care directives).
Organizational Ethics	A patient's trust in health care is based on trust in the ethical behavior of an individual physician.	An organization has moral standing and responsibility. Consumers and patients seek trust in organizational processes rather than simply in individuals.
Consumer Empowerment	A patient participates in decision making through informed consent for clinical decisions.	An organization informs consumers and patients of policies and rationales, encourages deliberation, and allows meaningful participation in policy decision making.

why the integration of organizational values with those of patients and doctors has made for a difficult marriage.

The active data-gathering phase of the BEST project entailed focused document collection, preliminary phone interviews, and two-day site visits to each of the participating health-care organizations. The site visits were in many ways the culminating feature of our pragmatic approach, in which we sought to reflect on realities in the field in conjunction with ethical theory. Our site visits were, of necessity, far ranging. We needed to understand the history of the organization, its place in the health-care market, and how the characteristics of that particular market helped shape the ethical world view of the organization. We needed to know what the baseline state regulations and legislative mandates were that framed what was minimally expected of any comparable health-care organization. We needed to understand not just *how* certain programs and policies functioned but *why*: Why had they decided to create a new appeals process from scratch two years ago? Why had they decided to redesign their confidentiality policies? Why had they shifted emphasis in their community benefit from outreach health programs to research support? Why did their organizational ethics program not create a code of ethics? These were the types of questions we needed to ask in order to investigate further the stories we were told and learn some of the deeper lessons about how organizations manage ethical tensions in a competitive environment.

Our site visits were also opportunities to seek corroborating evidence from multiple perspectives. If the CEO of a health plan touted her organization's medical policy programs we had to talk to as many people as possible to find out if the story rang true. We were not on a witch hunt to uncover conspiracies of deceptive or fraudulent conduct. But we know that it is inevitable that individuals and organizations wish to put the best light on their achievements. The concept of a site visit by itself is enough to throw some health-care organizations into a nearly operatic mode of self-aggrandizement. We had to listen carefully, ask many questions, and talk to many different sources to gain a deeper understanding of the programs, policies, and procedures in which we would be looking for exemplary practices.

DEFINING EXEMPLARY ETHICAL PRACTICES

An early concern of the participating organizations—one quite understandable given the acronym for the project—was the idea that the goal of the BEST project was to identify single *best* ethical practices. Unfortunately, in the current health-care environment, ethics is too easily held up as yet one more potential report-card evaluation in which any study of ethical practices evokes visions of judgmental measures of moral worth. In other words, if there is a *best* ethical practice, everyone else must be somehow deficient, and the underlying purpose of looking for rare examples of ethical excellence must be to uncover the many unethical failures. But a pragmatic approach favors the belief that there is rarely just one way of doing things that can be considered ethical. There are some approaches that may in fact be unethical because they violate or ignore central ethical values. More typically, however, there is a range of possible approaches to problems, all of which may be deemed ethically justifiable.

Within the organizational ethical domains we defined, every organizational policy and every tough decision and communication with patient and provider must address competing ethical values of true worth; consequently, there will be many ways to balance these values and realize an ethical outcome. For example, in making decisions about coverage of new medical treatments that have undergone limited evaluation, adherents of the major approaches to ethics and justice will all recognize certain sets of patient-centered and population-centered values as valid. Patient-centered values include giving proper attention to important patient needs, avoiding harms that can arise from adversarialism, and managing uncertainties and risks through collaborative treatment planning. Population-centered values include prudent use of shared resources (stewardship) and promotion of public goods such as knowledge about efficacy and safety. Any ethical approach to making coverage decisions, whether arising from utilitarian, deontological, principlist, or some other background, will find patient-centered and population-centered values as valid. But although these values will be universally accepted, reasonable persons will differ over how to weight and prioritize them in the context of specific decisions. Thus, difficult decisions regarding "experimental" therapies cannot be submitted to some canonical decision rule. The normative emphasis shifts away from the outcome of the decisions made and casts a stronger light instead upon the elements of the decision-making process (Daniels and Sabin, 1997).

But our analysis was not pragmatic in the sense that it accepted as ethical any policy or program that seemed to work. Nor were we satisfied with laying out minimal ethical requirements which would be easily met. In line with our overarching goal of moving the ethical bar higher and showing organizations various ways to reach it, we first developed general criteria for identifying *exemplary* ethical practices to address the ethical tensions within all of the domains we had identified. Our general criteria included the following:

- There is a coherent formulation of an organizational problem or challenge that reflects an awareness of conflicting values. The organization does not have to conceptualize the problem as an *ethical* issue, since for many executives, conflicting values or interests are not necessarily labeled *ethics*.
- There is a plan of considered action to manage the ethical tension that addresses the value conflicts. This plan must embody a way of specifying and balancing key ethical values, and reasons should be articulated for why the approach taken is the best way to realize an appropriate balance of values.

- There is a set of consistently applied procedures that are integrated into the organizations' functioning and that constitute a plausible means of implementing the process for managing the conflict of ethical values.
- There is a mechanism to evaluate the effectiveness of the implementation in meeting objectives. Such mechanisms might include internal or external audits, feedback from stakeholders, or collection of other data. If the organizational approach to managing the ethical tensions has existed for several years, there should be evidence of evaluation and subsequent modifications to enhance its effectiveness.

Having developed these general criteria for exemplary ethical practices, we went further to articulate specific normative obligations for exceptional performance within each of the ethical domains. These ethical obligations apply directly to the specific actions and decisions that arise in each domain, but the obligations are still broadly framed with the expectation that there are different ways in which an organization could achieve each goal. For example, in the domain of medical necessity, coverage decisions, and medical policy, one of our central ethical obligations holds that changes in benefits that reduce coverage or limit therapeutic options should include provisions to protect those patients at greatest risk. This is a normative obligation that prioritizes a specific ethical value, sets a clear goal, and provides a criterion with which to judge organizational benefit policy. But it does not dictate the specific means by which vulnerable patients should be protected. The aim of the site visits was to find good examples of innovative methods that organizations had developed to meet this kind of ethical obligation.

During the site visits and further analyses of the BEST organizations, our list of central ethical obligations for each domain did not remain static; it evolved in a dialectic fashion as we learned how the ethical dilemmas faced by each organization differed as a function of the organization's particular history, organizational structure, and market environment. Despite these differences, our final set of ethical obligations for each domain, which we present separately in the chapters that follow, reflect those obligations that we believe are the hallmark of all exemplary organizational efforts to manage the inherent ethical tensions they face.

Neither our general criteria for exemplary ethical practices nor the specific ethical obligations for each domain require that an organizational approach to value conflicts be sophisticated in any academic sense. Such an approach simply has to address the identified ethical tension in a manner that holds legitimacy for all stakeholders. Operating within the boundaries established by our central ethical obligations, that legitimacy rests upon an organization's public justification of both specific decisions and broader policy approaches through reasons that weigh relevant facts and values (Daniels and Sabin, 2002). Within this framework there is clearly room for more than one exemplary practice in an ethical domain. Indeed, for any given domain, different organizations, depending on the organizations' unique circumstances and culture, will create polices that seem to favor particular values. For example, one organization's policy on confidentiality might emphasize a member's absolute right of privacy while the policy of another might balance privacy with an emphasis on using records to enhance disease management.

The aim of the ethical analyses that we present in the following chapters is to describe distinctive approaches in each domain, identifying common themes and important differences in how the value conflicts are managed. From these distinctions, and from the lessons that we take from them, we aim to provide health-care organizations, policy makers, consumers, and others alternative road maps to enhancing ethical performance. Having started with a pragmatic approach to identifying the ethical challenges of health-care organizations, we used ethical theory to develop a framework of normative criteria to identify exemplary responses. Underpinned by extensive review of documents, in-depth interviews with key informants, and a concerted effort to gather information from the broad perspectives of all major stakeholders, the ethical analyses we present in the following chapters return us to our pragmatic goal by reflecting on theory in the light of experience and by comparing and contrasting various real-world approaches to managing the deepest ethical challenges faced by health-care organizations.

3

ORGANIZATIONAL ETHICS

> The newly designated fifty-first state—the island of Utopia—set out to reform its health-care system. The Secretary of Health and Happiness identified Utopia's most brilliant thinkers and convened a working group to determine the ethical characteristics of an ideal system. The island's luminaries produced an ethical code of dazzling clarity, admired by all who read it. It was published in Utopia's leading periodicals and featured on Utopian Public Radio. Unfortunately, a follow-up study of the code several years later showed that, while still referred to with respect, it had achieved no practical results.
>
> At about the same time, in the newly designated fifty-second state—the adjoining island of Pragmatica—an idealistic employee of Hardnosed Health Plan proposed creation of an organizational ethics program. He presented the idea to his boss. Her response was unambiguous. "Come on, get real! 'Ethics' is just a word. The French said it all years ago—'*Chacun a son gout.*' Ethics is personal. We do have to follow the dumb laws our legislature is always passing, but we should let the market sort out all the rest. Didn't you learn that at business school? Where do you think you are—Utopia?"

Organizational ethics is a new frontier for health-care ethics. Even if the United States moved from a system based on competing insurance companies to a single payer model or an individual voucher system, organizations—albeit different ones than in the market-driven managed care approach—would still be central determinants of the ethical quality of medical care. Managed care has dramatized the need for ethical standards for organizations, but it has not created this need.

Delivery of leading-edge, technically advanced health care typically depends on tertiary hospitals, research centers, and other complex enterprises. And, at the other pole of the health-care spectrum, population-oriented primary care and preventive medicine requires its own form of organizational infrastructure. Thus, the two poles of medical care—public-health-oriented primary care on the one hand, and sophisticated technological medicine on the other—both require organizations for their provision.

This should not come as a surprise. Thirty years ago, in the first sentence of his classic text on management, Peter Drucker wrote that "[d]uring the last fifty years, society in every developed country has become a society of institutions" (Drucker,

1973). But because most health care ultimately involves hands-on, person-to-person contact—with a doctor, nurse, physical therapist, or nursing home aide—health professionals and the U.S. public have only recently recognized how relevant Drucker's prescient vision is for the health sector.

Although business ethics is now taught at virtually every school of business, debate still rages between exponents of the invisible hand and the impassioned heart. On behalf of the invisible hand, Milton Friedman argues that "there is one and only one social responsibility of business—to use its resources and engage in activities designed to increase its profits" (Friedman, 1962). More recently, James Collins and Jerry Porras have countered by identifying "core values and purpose"— the impassioned heart—as the motivating force of successful enterprises (Collins and Porras, 1996).

Despite the ongoing debate, the contending parties largely agree that the distinctively human "product" in health care requires an organizational ethic that stipulates more than avoidance of illegal competitive practices and fraud (Ozar et al., 2000). It is easy, however, to preach the importance of ethics for health-care organizations, but much harder to clarify the substance of *organizational ethics* and to specify how organizations can best pursue this noble objective. That is the challenge for this chapter and a central purpose of our entire project.

Health-care organizational ethics has three interrelated but distinctive dimensions. The first is articulation of a moral compass for the organization, typically referred to as *mission, vision,* or *values.* Establishing and espousing the moral compass is a central task for organizational leaders. For this inspirational component of organizational ethics, the CEO must take the role of Chief Ethics Officer. The second element is more analytical—the ability to identify the ethical challenges that arise for the organization and address the inevitable conflicts among basic values—"good versus good"—in a systematic manner. This is the deliberative side of organizational ethics. Last, but in no way least, a robust organizational ethics must include management processes that lead to doing the right thing. Vision statements and moral deliberation that do not result in more worthy performance are at best a waste of time and resources and at worst, a duplicitous effort to clothe organizational wolves in the clothing of ethical sheep. High moral pronouncements without follow-through lead to distrust and cynicism. This practical, quality-improvement phase completes the organizational ethics cycle.

The word *ethics* is like a Rorschach inkblot—it elicits different meanings for different observers. For some, *ethics* refers to conduct, standards, and values. *Ethics* understood this way is easy to see as a relevant part of organizational life. For others, however, *ethics* connotes politically correct pieties that are irrelevant to real world action. For them, referring to *ethics* may be expedient, but the concept carries no force other than its public relations impact. And there are yet others for whom ethics is a routine expectation of responsible clinicians, managers, and organizations. Since they regard ethical conduct as standard operating procedure, they take offense at the idea that any special ethics activities are needed.

An organization that clearly understands its mission, identifies and manages conflicts among key values, and ensures that it acts in accord with these values, can be an exemplar of organizational ethics without using the word *ethics* for any of its operations.

BACKGROUND

Hospital Ethics Committees

The strongest and most direct precedent for the newly emerging *organizational* ethics activities is the 25-year history of hospital based *clinical* ethics committees and programs (Moreno, 1995). While there is much controversy about the role and effectiveness of these initiatives, they have established widely recognized examples of ways in which ethics can contribute to clinical functions in the hospital. The experience of hospital ethics committees and programs lends credence to the idea that managed care organizations and public sector health agencies may benefit from similar initiatives. And, since virtually all of the most widely respected hospitals have active ethics programs, the hospital experience creates an element of expectation that all exemplary health care organizations involved in managed care should follow a comparable path.

The accumulated national experience with hospital ethics committees provides health-care organizational ethics with a legacy of three main elements. First, the hospital precedent gives plausibility to the belief that careful attention to values and conflict among values has the potential to enhance organizational function and that ethics is not simply an academic or touchy-feely enterprise. Second, by including social workers, clergy, representatives of the public and others, hospital ethics committees have fostered broader stakeholder participation than had previously been typical in the medical sector. Finally, in a medical culture characterized by deep faith in scientific certainty and data-driven decision making, hospital ethics committees have created an element of legitimacy for moral deliberation as a respectable component of a science-based culture (Gutmann and Thompson, 1997).

As hospital-based clinical ethics programs accumulated experience and matured in the 1990s, committee members and friendly critics challenged them to progress beyond deliberation and education to a commitment to making measurable differences in patient care. In response, programs have taken a leaf from the quality improvement movement and asked how ethics can be integrated into the hospital's "production processes." Ethics consultants have adapted the clinical concepts of prevention and health promotion to ethics consultation, leading to an emphasis on "upstream" interventions aimed at preventing the kinds of ethical conundrums that ultimately came to ethics committees (Forrow et al., 1993). Some ethics committees have revised their mode of operation to emphasize a proactive effort to improve patient care by improving the ethical quality of hospital operations (Blake, 2000). The common theme of this push for change from within the world of hospital ethics programs is an effort to ensure that ethics activities achieve meaningful impact on organizational function and a belief that this can best be accomplished by integration with the organization, not by standing apart as an independent, but impotent, voice of conscience.

In 1995 the Joint Commission for Accreditation of Health Care Organizations (JCAHO)—the primary hospital accreditation organization in the United States—added a strong external push to this effort to link ethics to organizational function by extending its existing standards for patients rights and ethics to include new requirements for "organization ethics." JCAHO defines ethics as part of quality improvement: [T]he goal of the patient rights and organization ethics function is to help improve patient outcomes" (JCAHO, 2002, p. 67). While the standards require a code of ethical behavior, they ask that "guiding documents, such as the hospital's mission statement and strategic plan, provide a consistent, ethical framework for its patient care and business practices" (JCAHO, 2002, p. 79). The standards specifically require that "regardless of how the hospital compensates or shares financial risk with its leaders, managers, clinical staff, and licensed independent practitioners," it must "protect the integrity of clinical decision making" (JCAHO, 2002, p. 80).

Between the 25-year legacy of hospital ethics committees and the more recent JCAHO standards for rights and organizational ethics, hospitals provide a strong precedent for seeing health-care organizations as agents whose ethical conduct influences the health of those it serves. From this perspective, concern about ethics is part of a fundamental concern with quality, not an add-on. Without specifying what must be done, JCAHO asks for ethics to be part of the organization's standard operating procedures.

Compliance Programs

Law, like ethics, is concerned with what we should and should not do. Corporate compliance programs, which are designed to prevent unlawful conduct and to promote conformity with externally imposed regulations, provide a second component of background for organizational ethics. Compliance programs came to prominence in the 1980s in the wake of widely publicized defense industry scandals. In health care, recurrent investigations of Medicare and Medicaid fraud and abuse have had the same impact on the emergence of compliance programs.

Compliance programs received a tremendous boost in 1991, when federal sentencing guidelines, which are designed to create consistency of sentencing in federal courts, allowed for reduced penalties for corporations convicted of federal violations if the company had implemented compliance initiatives that met seven sensible standards. To protect itself against maximum penalties, an organization must have placed a high-level person in charge of procedures "reasonably capable of reducing the prospect of criminal conduct"; appropriate training, monitoring, enforcement, and corrective responses to any offenses must occur; and the organization must be diligent in its hiring and delegation practices (Dubinsky, 1997).

The evolving field of health-care organizational ethics has had a love/hate relationship with compliance. Compliance is about meeting legal and regulatory requirements, and the activity is often led by lawyers. The basic question for compliance is "What are we required to do?" Health-care ethics is largely about patient care, and the activity is often led by clinically oriented managers or clinicians. The basic question for ethics is "What is the right thing to do?" Compliance, in its narrowest construction, is about obedience or *avoiding guilt*. Ethics, in its narrowest construction, is about self-governance or *pursuing virtue*.

Serious attention to law and regulation and to ethical obligations are potentially synergistic activities. If compliance and ethics are defined narrowly as avoiding guilt and pursuing virtue, they will be difficult to integrate. Some leading theorists, however, are beginning to conceptualize the two activities as different facets of organizational integrity and suggest that there may be advantages to both in bringing compliance and ethics together (Mills and Spencer, 2001). Because compliance programs help organizations reduce the risk of severe penalties, they receive strong endorsement from boards and top management. Compliance programs are seen as mandatory, not optional. They are at risk, however, of being viewed by staff as a way for the corporation and its leaders to protect themselves and not as connected to important care values. Ethics programs, by contrast, are devoted to important values but may be seen as optional, even if worthy.

In principle, compliance and ethics can complement each other. Compliance brings attention to the details of performance and enforcement power. Ethics taps staff ideals and brings attention to deliberation and analysis. A partnership between the two activities could be stronger than having two independent programs.

Commissions and Codes

At the same time that federal and state legislation sought to create a framework of expectations for organizational conduct in the managed care arena, ethicists sought to do the same thing from the perspective of ethics. Since ethics codes have no official status and no penalties for not following them, none of the work on ethics codes has had the same immediate impact on organizational compliance that legislation and regulation have produced. We discuss below the reports of four commissions in order to suggest the contours of ethical reflection—two were developed by regional ethics centers and two by national professional organizations. Our aim here is to highlight the central practical implications for the ethics of organizations, not to summarize the details of the four reports.

In 1994, the Midwest Bioethics Center, with support from the Kansas City-based Prime Health Foundation, set out "to improve the quality of health care . . . by *supporting* a culture of ethical sensitivity and behavior in managed care organizations" (Biblo et al., 1996). "Ethical issues in managed care," published in 1996, is laden with specific recommendations (127 numbered suggestions), but it contains a crisp core vision. The report identifies resource allocation as the overriding ethical issue in managed care. It recommends pursuing "the well-being of the entire group for whom the decisions are being made, balanced by the requirement to respect individual health care needs" as the ethical compass for managed care organizations. It sees a corporate "culture where ethical considerations are integrated into decision making at all levels" as the key requirement for improved ethical performance. It concludes that to support a culture of ethics, organizations must orchestrate deliberative processes in which health plans, providers, and members seek a justifiable balance among multiple values.

In 1998, after a two-year process that involved 700 consumers, patients, providers, employers, and health plan representatives, the Rocky Mountain Center for Healthcare Ethics published the *Colorado Code of Ethics for Healthcare*.[1] While the code has no official status, the inclusion of leaders of Colorado's professional societies, health plans, provider associations, business groups, and Department of Public Health on the steering committee, combined with a robust dissemination process, have given it wide visibility in the state. The code contains seven principles, each introduced by a value statement, followed by standards that "delineate behavioral expectations for the ethical delivery and reception of healthcare."

Of greatest salience for organizational ethics, Colorado identifies the goal of health care as "maximiz[ing] the health of individuals and populations" and states that "regardless of the competitive environment, participants collaborate to improve the health of the public." It identifies "appropriate" use of resources as a responsibility for consumers and patients, as well as health plans and payers. And, like the report from the Midwest Bioethics Center, it emphasizes that "ethical tensions and conflicts are inevitable" and calls on participants in health care to "work individually and collectively to identify and seek to resolve ethical concerns."

In 1999 the Institute for Ethics at the American Medical Association (AMA) convened a working group on organizational ethics, whose work was published in 2000 as *Organizational Ethics in Healthcare: Toward a Model for Ethical Decision Making by Provider Organizations* (Ozar et al., 2000). The AMA publishes and regularly updates a widely used code of medical ethics for physicians, so developing a code for provider organizations was a natural next step. The purpose of the resulting scholarly essay is first to determine, on the basis of existing ethical systems, what should count as ethical conduct for provider organizations and then to propose a model for ethical decision making. A particular strength of the essay is that it identifies ethical areas in which there is no national consensus. The authors deliberately leave these areas unresolved. Thus, after identifying patients' health as the highest priority for provider organizations, the essay notes that there is little public agreement on how health itself should be understood, and even less agreement on how trade-offs between the interests of different patient populations should be made. A second strength of the essay is that, after a scholarly analysis, it offers a fictional but highly detailed case to which it applies its methodology. The case discussion, like Harry Truman's one-armed economist, avoids the "on the one hand/on the other hand" trap and reaches a well-argued conclusion, suggesting that the decision-making model can be applied in practice.

Finally, in 2000, with support from the Open Society Institute's Medicine as a Profession program, the American College of Physicians/American Society of Internal Medicine convened a working group of clinicians, consumers, ethicists, managed care insurers, and purchasers to develop ethical guidelines for managed care. In the spring of 2001 the 16-member group completed *Ethics in Practice: Managed Care and the Changing Health Care Environment.*[2] By the fall of 2001, 12 organizations, representing patients (American Diabetes Association, Citizen Advocacy Center), physicians (American Academy of Pediatrics, American Association of Public Health Physicians) and accreditation (National Committee for Quality Assurance), had formally endorsed the statement.

The American College of Physicians/American Society of Internal Medicine statement includes four principles, amplified as 21 subprinciples. Of most importance for the ethics of health-care organizations, the statement treats organizations as if they were individuals, subject to the same conceptions of virtue and the same kinds of moral accountabilities. Thus when principle IA states that "health plans, purchasers, clinicians and patients should be open and truthful in their dealings with each other," it is envisioning a dialogue between three parties in which all should comport themselves by the same ethical standard. Similarly, principle II and IIA treat organizations as morally accountable beings by stating that "[h]ealth plans, purchasers, clinicians and the public share responsibility for the appropriate stewardship of health care resources . . . [and] should take part in a public dialogue shaping policies on the quality of and access to care."

None of the four statements of codes and principles has official standing or any power of enforcement. All contain excellent, sensible ethical recommendations, and there is a great deal of consistency among the statements, but to the best of our knowledge, none hasve been used in a formal way as a guide to action by any actual organization. The lesson from the experience in ethical code development from 1994 until the present is that, as important as statements of ethical principles may be, developing a code has little traction in itself, notwithstanding the prestige of the body promulgating it. Organizations do not appear to be looking for codes and principles. This does not mean that organizations are unethical. It may be that codes, per se, are not answering a question that organizations are asking.

ETHICAL VALUES AND CENTRAL ETHICAL OBLIGATIONS

In health care, values permeate every component of organizational activity. We expect that there are many pathways by which organizations can consistently and reliably act with integrity over time. We do not believe that any specific form of mission statement, ethics committee, or management process is a necessary prerequisite for ethical organizational conduct. But we do believe that an ethically admirable organization must meet three core challenges: Ethically admirable organizations must have a deeply held set of values appropriate to care of the sick and promotion of health, they must be skillful at dealing with the values conflicts that inevitably arise in health care, and they must make sure that they live by their values.

We use the term *organizational ethics* to refer to the organization's efforts to *define* its own core values and mission, *identify* areas in which important values come into conflict, *seek* the best possible resolution of these conflicts, and *manage* its own performance to ensure that it acts in accord with espoused values. We do not assume that these activities will necessarily be called *ethics*. The goal of organizational ethics is to enable the enterprise to conduct itself with integrity in the full range of its activities. To assess organizational ethics, we examine the clarity and effectiveness with which the organization pursues each of the different components.

Our approach to organizational ethics focuses primarily on ethical *procedures*. As described in the preceding chapter, we do not postulate a single normative template for assessing the ethics of health-care organizations. All health-care organizations work within some form of resource limits, and within the U.S. version of managed care, all must face the stringencies of market competition. All must address the challenge of how to set priorities and enforce limits in a way that is clinically sound, ethically justifiable, and politically acceptable. If there were consensus on fine-grained principles of distributive justice, these principles would provide a template for all organizations. But since pluralistic societies have no such consensus (Daniels and Sabin, 1997), we take a pragmatic approach that emphasizes broad normative values and the elements of a procedural justice that create legitimacy for difficult decisions. Our list of central ethical obligations for exemplary performance in organizational ethics is shown in Table 3–1.

Table 3–1. Central ethical obligations for organizational ethics

AN EXEMPLARY ETHICAL ORGANIZATION MUST:

1. Hold deeply a set of values emphasizing care of the sick and the promotion of health.
2. Involve key stakeholders in identifying its values and in managing value conflicts.
3. State clearly and forcefully those values it commits itself to and guides itself by.
4. Disseminate understanding of its values to its entire staff.
5. Recognize that the full range of its activities influences the ethical quality of patient care.
6. Cultivate skill at identifying threats to and conflicts among its values.
7. Deliberate about value conflicts in light of what it has done and learned in previous similar conflict situations.
8. Ensure that it acts on its values: It "walks the walk" as well as "talks the talk."
9. Partner only with others who live by compatible values.

EXEMPLARY PRACTICES

Organizational Ethics through Compliance— Foundation Health Plan of Florida

Foundation Health Plan of Florida is the Florida component of Health Net, a national for-profit managed care company.[3] Its corporate ethos is the belief that the surest path to efficient, cost-effective care is rigorous pursuit of quality. With evidence-based quality of care as *the* guiding value for the enterprise, Foundation Health sees no role for an independent organizational ethics function.

Foundation Health could support its approach to organizational ethics by citing the AMA report *Organizational Ethics in Healthcare*, (Ozar et al., 2000) which identified patients' health as *the* preeminent value in health care. If patients' health is *the* prime value for health care, and a focus on quality is *the* primary road for promoting that goal, what could an organizational ethics program be but a frill or a distraction? From this perspective, the only values that require special managerial attention other than quality of care are the values embodied in state and federal regulatory requirements. These requirements reflect the values the public has chosen to promote through governmental activity. For Foundation Health of Florida, clinical quality management and corporate compliance are the means for seeking to be an ethical organization.

For corporate compliance programs, regulatory requirements provide the equivalent of a code of ethics. Given that regulations are identical for all organizations of the same kind in the same geographical area, organizations cannot be exemplary on the basis of the values their compliance programs pursue since the source of these values is the same external regulations all must meet. Foundation Health of Florida's approach to compliance is distinguished by four elements: the diligence with which it identifies external requirements, the distinctive way it educates its staff, the way it responds to defects, and its attitude towards disclosure.

All organizations subject to regulations face penalties if they do not adhere to the regulations. There is, however, a broad spectrum of responses, ranging from slow, grudging compliance with the letter of the law in a minimalist fashion to proactive interaction with regulatory agencies, aimed at understanding the spirit as well as the letter of regulatory law as a basis for organizational action.

Although relatively small by industry standards, Foundation Health of Florida devotes the major component of a staff position to intense, often daily, communication with the Florida Division of Insurance and Office of Personnel, the federal Medicare office, and other regulatory bodies. The aim is to translate regulatory objectives into staff education and internal monitoring systems.

The risk of basing organizational ethics on compliance is that an ethic based on prohibitions ("thou shalt not . . .") is unlikely to elicit the same kind of positive motivations as an ethic based on ideals ("thou shalt . . ."). For that reason, Foundation Health of Florida seeks to understand and explain compliance requirements in the light of the positive aims (ideals) they embody: Accurate claims information embodies honesty. Timely claims payment treats providers with respect. Abandoned telephone calls represent members who are—figuratively speaking—sent away when they seek help. When we asked the compliance director how staff saw the program, she responded, "50% as ethics and 50% as policing." Achieving a 50% perception as "ethics" for a compliance program is a substantial achievement for corporate compliance!

Foundation Health of Florida develops audit standards to monitor compliance with regulations. Thus, with regard to claims processing, the organization monitors activities like entry of claims information in an ongoing way. Even if standards are being met, a dip in performance allows the compliance team to ask why this has happened. Compliance is wedded to the quality improvement methodology of monitoring production processes and reengineering when needed.

Quality improvement teaches that "every defect is a treasure," and *realpolitik* teaches that cover-ups ultimately return to haunt the concealer. Foundation Health of Florida follows a policy of disclosure of failures of compliance. That policy reflects ideals ("Disclosure is the right thing to do"), pragmatic considerations ("Disclosure encourages the regulators to trust us"), and pride in accomplishment ("We have been doing so well it is not embarrassing when we miss the mark").

Foundation Health of Florida's approach to corporate compliance shows that compliance programs can be stretched to encompass at least some of the mission-setting, inspirational component of organizational ethics as well as the performance-monitoring component that compliance is designed to achieve. By emphasizing the human values that dry, bureaucratic regulations are aimed at promoting and by linking compliance to the broad corporate commitment to quality, Foundation Health of Florida moves compliance well beyond avoiding guilt in the direction of pursuing virtue.

Organizational Ethics through Deliberation— Harvard Pilgrim Health Care

Foundation Health of Florida focused its approach to organizational ethics on the effort to ensure that the organization acted on its values. It derived those values from two sources—the commitment to evidence-based quality, and laws and regulations. It located its equivalent of an ethics endeavor within the corporate compliance area. By contrast, Harvard Pilgrim Health Care (HPHC) made cultivation of skill at identifying stakeholder values and deliberation about the best way to respond to conflicts among these values the basis of its approach to organizational ethics. Accordingly, it chose to develop an independent organizational ethics program separate from the compliance function.

Before the HPHC ethics program was launched in 1996, one of its two precursor organizations—Harvard Community Health Plan—vacillated for more than a decade over whether or not to do it. A task force on "humanistic health care" in the 1970s was perceived as having become a nonconstructive forum for complaint, and the management feared that an ethics program might follow the same route. In the 1980s, managers feared that an ethics program might inadvertently take accountability for grappling with ethical problems away from the responsible program managers. It was only after the 1995 merger of Harvard Community Health Plan, founded as a not-for-profit, staff-model health maintenance organization, with Pilgrim Health Care, a not-for-profit, independent-practice association, that the new organization decided to create an ethics program.

HPHC finally settled its ambivalence about creating an ethics program for three main reasons. First, although both partners to the merger were widely respected in the local community as highly ethical not-for-profit organizations, the cultures of values in the two organizations were distinctive enough that each feared that the other might contain "unethical" elements. Second, the external environment had moved away from community rating and was creating ever stronger pressure for cost reductions. The organization saw these environmental changes as major ethical challenges. Finally, the medical director and CEO were both enthusiastic about the idea. They announced the new program as follows:

> Each day, it seems we are bombarded with stories raising public awareness of the basic tension at the heart of the health care debate: namely that of preserving a health care system which fundamentally supports the best interests of individual patients while balancing society's need to ensure affordable, accessible, quality health care for an entire population within a finite amount of resources. . . . The goals of the Ethics Program are to:

- Promote increased organizational skill at identifying and explicitly addressing the ethical dimensions of key policy, operational and budgetary decisions.
- Establish and support an educational program to assure knowledge, skills, and competence in facilitating ethical decision making.
- Demonstrate to our members and purchasers that Harvard Pilgrim Health Care is actively concerned with ethical and quality issues. . . .
- Assure that Harvard Pilgrim Health Care is prepared to address the ethical aspects of issues being forced by our competitive market with confidence that our processes withstand public scrutiny.
- Attain national recognition as managed care leaders in this initiative.

The CEO and medical director appointed Lisa Raiola as founding director of the HPHC ethics programs. Although Ms. Raiola majored in biomedical ethics as an undergraduate at Brown, her primary work experience had been in strategic planning, human resources, and organizational development. In retrospect, her skills in these areas were crucial for the development of the program.

Ms. Raiola began by interviewing all members of the senior leadership and the board of directors to get their views about the central ethical issues facing the organization and the best way to develop an organizational ethics program. The HPHC board and leadership believed that positioning the program as a consultative function with no "must approve" role would decrease fear of the new venture and facilitate its use. With their encouragement, she defined the program as a "decision-support" function with no administrative authority, and formed an Ethics Advisory Group as the hub of the ethics program.

The Ethics Advisory Group is the most distinctive feature of the HPHC approach to organizational ethics. The group is composed of HPHC's key stakeholders—staff, HPHC members ("consumers"), physicians from the HPHC network, purchasers, and representatives of the public. In accord with the decision to make the ethics program a consultative, decision-support activity, the group only addresses issues that are brought to it by a manager—referred to as the *customer*—who is responsible for the area in question.

The Ethics Advisory Group meeting on June 30, 1997, marked the program's coming of age. The customer for that meeting was the CEO, who asked for consultation about a rapidly unfolding series of events about which he had to make an immediate, highly visible decision. Five pediatricians from the former staff-model segment of the organization had resigned as a group to set up their own pediatric group practice. They applied for membership in the HPHC network, which would allow them to take patients from the staff-model program with them. They would be in direct competition with the former staff-model practice.

The CEO was facing a classical "good vs. good" conflict. The pediatricians were popular, and it was anticipated that many families would leave the staff-model practice to continue with them. At the same time, the staff model practice felt that the departing pediatricians were not entitled to take with them a panel of patients that had been developed through the staff model, when doing so would deprive the staff model of membership and capitation payments. Continuity of care and patient choice were important values, but so was the integrity of the staff-model practice. A June 18 *Boston Globe* article was headlined "Doctor's departure shakes up HMO," putting the CEO's decision under an intense public spotlight.

The Ethics Advisory Group reviewed the facts of the situation and considered which values should be preeminent. Noting that HPHC defined as its mission "improving the health of the people we serve," it found that the most important value in the case was continuity of care and patient preference. From this perspective, no barriers should be put in the way of allowing patients to continue with their caretakers. But in light of the HPHC vision of "being the most trusted and respected name in health care," the Ethics Advisory Group identified the integrity of the staff-model practice as another a key value. It advised that, while the pediatricians were entitled to request membership in the HPHC network, receiving network membership was not an entitlement.

The CEO made his decision in accord with the consultation. Members who wanted to continue with the departing pediatricians were given insurance coverage to do so for the remainder of their insurance contract year. The departing pediatricians, however, were not allowed to join the HPHC network. Members would ultimately have to decide whether they wanted to take new insurance, which would allow them to continue with their pediatricians. The CEO felt that this course of action best protected the organization's key values. Since continuity of care was the leading value in the situation, members were not forced to make an immediate choice between continuing with their pediatricians or switching to other staff-model pediatricians. But supporting the staff-model practice was also important, and not inviting the pediatricians to join the HPHC network supported that value. Physicians would not be allowed to build up a practice and then steal that practice from the group.

In 2001, HPHC reviewed the first five years of experience with its ethics program. It assessed the consultative and decision-support functions as a resounding success. The multistakeholder Ethics Advisory Group had clearly emerged as a respected deliberative and advisory body. Minutes from the meetings were posted on the staff and provider websites and were read widely.

The review identified two areas for potential improvement. First, the program had initially focused its attention on difficult decisions for which it provided consultation through the Ethics Advisory Group. In the course of providing more than 40 consultations, the group had developed considerable skill at responding to problems that had already surfaced. At the five-year point, HPHC's leadership asked the program to do more to help the organization anticipate future ethical challenges and plan for them. Second, the review concluded that the program's initial strategy of relying on education as the mechanism for enhancing HPHC's overall quality of ethical performance was too indirect. The kinds of classroom educational sessions that the ethics program had conducted were well received by participants, but it had been difficult for staff to connect the classroom experience to practical action.

As a result of the five-year review, the program shifted its structure. To make a better connection between organizational action and the insights that emerged from the deliberations of the Ethics Advisory Group, the new program director was asked to bring the perspectives of the ethics program to two operations groups—the member appeals committee, which heard and decided on appeals, and the benefit policy committee, which had responsibility for contract management and the development of new benefit policies. And to help the ethics program focus on planning for future ethical challenges, oversight of the program was shifted to the strategic development section of the organization. The intent was to make anticipatory ethical analysis part of the strategic planning process.

As part of the review process, the Ethics Advisory Group examined some of the proposed managed care ethics codes to see if the codes might help in its deliberative process. The group decided they did not. The problem was not disagreement with the content of the codes but a sense that, compared to starting by struggling with the values articulated by stakeholders who were in the room, deliberation based on codes felt removed from the texture and reality of the actual situation. The Ethics Advisory Group elected to retain its method of careful elucidation of stakeholder values, using codes as a kind of checklist for asking whether any important dimensions had been overlooked.

Organizational Ethics through Integrity—Holy Cross Health System

Holy Cross Health System, which became part of Trinity Health in 2000, was founded by the Sisters of the Holy Cross, a congregation originating in France, whose mission to the United States began in the 1860s. Its headquarters are in South Bend, Indiana, with member hospitals, residential care facilities, and community clinics in Maryland, Ohio, Indiana, Idaho, and California.

The organization states its mission in two powerful sentences:

> Faithful to the spirit of the Congregation of the Sisters of the Holy Cross, the Holy Cross Health System exists to witness Christ's love through excellence in the delivery of health services motivated by respect for those we serve. We foster a climate that empowers those who serve with us while stewarding our human and financial resources.

Our visits to several facilities in 1999 showed wide recognition of the mission statement. It was posted on office walls, printed on the back of individual business cards, and frequently cited by interviewees. Although the organization's mission is stated in terms of Christian theology, we interviewed non-Christian members of the staff as well. For them, the mission statement had meaning as a passionate commitment to caretaking values, not as a religiously derived truth. Although they did not share the theology of the mission, they did share the view of health care as a calling.

Holy Cross uses the mission statement as the basis of a comprehensive approach to organizational ethics that has two central components. The Organizational Integrity Program represents an effort to merge *compliance* with *ethics*; the Mission Discernment Process represents a frontal approach to making sure that the Holy Cross mission leads to action, not just words.

The first sentence of the 40-page booklet *Organizational Integrity Program*[4] sets forth the dual nature of the program:

> Holy Cross Health System is committed to complying with all ethical, professional and legal obligations, and to fostering a culture that enables all those associated with Holy Cross to fulfill these obligations.

The commitment is to comply with expectations, but the pathway towards achieving it is organizational culture, and the standards with which the system must comply are explicitly defined as ethical and professional as well as legal. The booklet goes on to explain the program as follows:

> This ongoing initiative is called an Integrity Program because it goes a step beyond traditional compliance programs that focus exclusively on conformity to law and the prevention of misconduct. The Integrity Program combines a concern for fulfilling the requirements of the law with an emphasis on responsible conduct, a renewed commitment to excellence and stewardship of resources, and a supportive work environment.

When we attended a meeting of the Organizational Integrity Council at a Holy Cross facility, we questioned the group about what going "a step beyond traditional compliance" actually meant. One participant responded, "More than just getting through the day without getting indicted . . . more than following rules and staying out of trouble . . . it is about the question 'What is the right thing to do?'" The leader of the council told us that the initial statement of standards had been written from a legal perspective. Staff responded negatively: "What is this all about? Why are we doing it?" Once traditional compliance was reconceptualized as a component of integrity and as part of the core mission, there was widespread acceptance. The Council leader concluded, "You can't give responsible people a task defined in terms of legal obligations and not expect them to want to re-craft it."

All Holy Cross staff are trained with regard to the expected standards of conduct. If they become aware of actual or potential violations or are concerned about what is right to do, they are honor-bound to follow a four step process: (*1*) Deal with the situation locally, including the possibility of contacting the immediate supervisor; (2) If not comfortable with or satisfied by local action, contact a higher level manager; (3) If still not satisfied, contact the local Integrity Officer; (4) If 1–3 have not resolved the concern, call the 24-hour Integrity Hot Line. The hot line is staffed by an outside organization and does not use Caller ID. Holy Cross commits itself to a policy that prohibits any form of retribution for good-faith reports of concerns.

The most distinctive component of the Holy Cross approach to organizational ethics is its Mission Discernment Process. Mission discernment is defined as part of the planning process that assesses new proposals in the light of the mission as well as through financial and operational analysis. As a rule of thumb, if a proposal will significantly affect the organization, its staff, stakeholders, or the community, mission discernment should be part of the planning process.[5] Holy Cross has developed a systematic list of questions that are discussed to determine the impact of major initiatives on meeting the ethical norms derived from the mission statement. The questions include: What considerations make this decision important for the mission and values of Holy Cross Health System? How will the quality of services be determined and maintained? How will care for the poor be addressed by this development? What is the community benefit from the project? The mission discernment process is not intended to yield a "yes" or "no" decision; rather, it is a process through which the organization investigates how the proposed policies or decisions can be restructured to best realize the mission.

At a site visit to Mount Carmel Medical Center in Columbus, Ohio, we sat in on a mission discernment meeting. The proposal being considered involved opening a new ambulatory care site integral to the medical center's expansion strategy. One aspect of the discussion focused on the fact that the neighborhood of the proposed site included a community of people with deafness. "Social justice for all" is a fundamental value for the organization, and a commitment to care for disadvantaged populations is a manifestation of that value. Questions were raised about how the proposed facility would accommodate the needs of patients with deafness, particularly the need for sign language interpreters. After much discussion, the new site was accepted on the condition that sign language interpretation for deaf patients would be made available.

LESSONS LEARNED

As a matter of national policy, the United States has largely eschewed comprehensive public debate about the values that should govern its health-care system. This national posture of head in the sand is largely motivated by the fact that serious discussion of health system values would require explicit recognition of limits. American political dialogue—with rare exceptions such as Oregon—prefers to pretend that, with regard to health care, there is a Santa Claus and that all our health-care needs and wishes can be fulfilled without sacrifice.

The national turn to a competitive system of managed care was based on a political hope that the invisible hand of the market would set limits in health-care expenditures without requiring political leaders to acknowledge and endorse what had to be done. To a significant degree, the intense public backlash against managed care reflects the predictable reaction of blaming the messenger for the message.

Thus, the three organizations featured in this chapter are seeking a moral compass within a political culture that deliberately avoids discussing the ethics of limits. Foundation Health of Florida, Harvard Pilgrim Health Care, and Holy Cross Health System can be seen as learning laboratories for addressing the two basic questions evoked at the opening of the chapter by the imaginary island states of Utopia and Pragmatica—where will the moral compass come from and how can it influence action? Not surprisingly for a society as pluralistic as the United States, the three organizations came up with decidedly different answers.

Foundation Health of Florida derived its approach to ethics from law and science. Although philosophers question whether ethics ("ought") can be derived from facts ("is"), in practical terms, that is exactly what Foundation Health did. Its implicit moral compass could be rendered as "Define insurance coverage in accord with scientific evidence, and conduct the organization in accord with law and regulation." Foundation Health of Florida steered itself by an empirically derived ethical compass.

Harvard Pilgrim Health Care bases its approach to organizational ethics on the quintessentially American doctrine of stakeholder theory. The Ethics Advisory Group explicitly seeks out the perspectives of the organization's key stakeholders—members ("consumers"), purchasers, clinicians, and organizational staff. The organization's vision of being "the most trusted and respected name in health care" emphasizes the bedrock importance of reliably meeting the core interests of its constituency. Its mission of "improving the health of the people we serve and the health of society," establishes health outcomes as the top priority among multiple stakeholder interests. Harvard Pilgrim's ethical compass emerges from the careful weighing and balancing of stakeholder values, with health outcomes given pride of place.

As a faith-based system, Holy Cross Health System grounds its approach to ethics on divinely revealed natural law by declaring that it "exists to witness Christ's love through excellence in the delivery of health services." While medicine is often characterized as a vocation or calling, and while the Hippocratic Oath has its origins in religious observation, only a faith-based organization is likely to be able to guide itself by natural law. Holy Cross's ethical compass is based on religious revelation and a view of medicine as a sacred calling. However, it is entirely possible for organizations guided by a secular vision to apply Holy Cross's concept of mission discernment to their own activities.

Although the three programs derive their approaches to organizational ethics from decidedly different sources, they have in common great clarity about the values they guide themselves by and intense commitment to realizing those values in action. The three organizational vignettes point toward a valuable practical lesson. They tell us that there are at least three distinctive ways to ground a health-care organization's approach to ethics. Unlike the mythical island state of Pragmatica, Foundation Health, Harvard Pilgrim, and Holy Cross were not skeptical about the need for a guiding ethic. But unlike the neighboring state of Utopia, they did not wait until society reached consensus about health-care ethics before taking action, the way the Utopians did. Instead, they each articulated and applied their own system of values. The stories of the three organizations suggest that improved ethical conduct by health-care organizations requires clarity about guiding values and determination to apply these values in action.

The second central challenge for organizational ethics—the one the state of Utopia discovered when its superbly crafted code of ethics produced no results—is the question of whether ethics can have real traction in organizational behavior. Our brief discussion of U.S. experience with four ethics codes developed for use in the managed care arena suggests that codes and principles in themselves accomplish little. Are there promising approaches to making ethics effective on the ground? The three organizational stories cited in this chapter, when combined with the chapters that follow, suggest an answer.

Mission statements, like ethics codes, provide the content for an organization's moral compass. But a compass cannot steer a ship by itself. The first step in making the mission statement have a real influence on the conduct of the organization is dissemination. Holy Cross Health System shows this especially clearly. The mission statement and its associated values are everywhere—on office walls, in organizational memos, on business cards, and more. But as necessary as broad dissemination is as a beginning step, the key question is not whether a statement of mission and values reads well or is posted on the walls, but whether leaders and managers actually use it in the daily life of the enterprise.

We think about the relationship between health-care organizations and those they serve in parallel to the relationship between physicians and their patients. For exemplary physicians, ethics is largely second nature. Seeking to understand their patients' values, planning treatment collaboratively, and—most importantly—caring deeply about their patients and conveying that caring in action is simply what they do. We ordinarily refer to this habitual behavior pattern as *character*, *virtue*, or, using the term that Holy Cross relies on, *integrity*.

By analogy, exemplary ethical organizations will conduct themselves with character, virtue, and integrity. The key lessons from the three organizations about how to do this are embarrassingly simple. To conduct themselves as ethical exemplars, organizations must espouse clear values. These values must be widely understood and shared throughout the organization. And, most importantly, leaders must be determined to apply these values in action consistently and reliably.

At this point, a skeptical reader may want to issue a challenge. "You are supposed to be talking about organizational ethics, but most of what you have discussed so far is about mission statements, committees, and management. Where does ethics come into the picture? What is the content of the ethics you are talking about?"

For enterprises like the ones we discuss in this and the subsequent chapters, organizational ethics is much more about the way the organization executes everyday actions than it is about making proclamations about how to balance individual and collective interests or whether health care is a right. Exemplary organizations put their greatest effort into putting their values into practice. The four elegant ethics codes discussed at the beginning of the chapter would answer the skeptical reader's request for content, but they have had extremely limited impact on action. They suffer from neglect, not from refutation.

Organizational ethics is a way of acting, not a code of principles. Foundation Health of Florida showed how the relatively meager ethical guidance provided by law and regulation could provide the basis for organizational control systems. Harvard Pilgrim Health Care uses its Ethics Advisory Group to elicit stakeholder perspectives on the organization's central ethical challenges, which then must be translated into useful guidance for operations. Holy Cross Health System, drawing on Catholic tradition of natural law, puts its values into action through the mission discernment process.

Organizational ethics remains a broad concept, one that encompasses culture, character, processes, and outcomes. In the chapters that follow, we will look carefully at ethical domains that are more focused and tightly linked to the structure and decision-making processes of health-care organizations. In many ways, however, all of the subsequent ethical domains we will discuss are problems for organizational ethics. How consumers are empowered; how medical necessity and coverage decisions are reached; how the care of vulnerable populations is integrated into the business structure of the organization; all these and other ethical questions find their first answers in the paradigm of organizational ethics held by an organization. Organizational ethics is thus a crucial framing attribute of health-care organizations in competitive markets. Within the body of an organization, organizational ethics is at the heart, pumping the blood that perfuses the entire organization with a common sense of purpose and a shared set of values. Without strong organizational ethics, a health-care organization in a competitive market cannot escape confusing the market as the source of its values and as the arbiter of value conflicts. We therefore place organizational ethics at the front of our work. It holds a primary lesson from the U.S. managed care experience: there are several paths to creating "good" organizations that can manage value conflicts in ethical, legitimate ways. How such organizations address the specific ethical problems they face in the marketplace is the subject to which we now turn.

NOTES

1. The Rocky Mountain Center for Healthcare Ethics was discontinued in 2000. The Colorado Code is now a project of the Center For Bioethics and Humanities (Richard Martinez, M.D., M.H.) Campus Box B-137, 4200 E. Ninth Avenue, Denver, CO 80262.

2. Available from Lois Snyder, JD, Center for Ethics and Professionalism, American College of Physicians-American Society of Internal Medicine, Philadelphia, PA 19106–1572.

3. In August 2001, two and a half years after our visit, Foundation Health Plan of Florida was sold to Vista Health Plan. Our references to corporate philosophy and practice apply to Foundation Health before its sale. To maintain consistency of style, however, we use the present tense in our discussion of Foundation Health.

4. *Organizational Integrity Program* (1997). Available from Holy Cross Health System, 3606 East Jefferson Boulevard, South Bend, IN 46615–3097.

5. *Mission Discernment: A Corporate Reflection Process* (1997). Available from Holy Cross Health System, 3606 East Jefferson Boulevard, South Bend, IN 46615–3097.

4

CONSUMER EMPOWERMENT

Safecare, a managed care plan, announced that it was pulling out of Medicare in a particular county. Safecare had sustained significant financial losses during the last three years, and the announcement stated that Medicare reimbursement was inadequate to cover the cost of providing care to patients in that county. Those long-term members of Safecare who were now over 65 and enrolled through Medicare learned that the plan they had belonged to for more than 30 years was dropping their coverage. The members who were threatened with loss of the plan as a group and wrote a petition to the organization: "We have been loyal and committed members for up to 30 years. If Safecare leaves our county, some of us will lose longstanding doctor relationships. How can Safecare have made this decision without even giving us a chance to influence it beforehand?"

The city of Philadelphia was determined to unify its Medicaid-supported substance abuse and mental health services into an innovative, city-wide managed care system. But bold ideas in the public mental health sector—like deinstitutionalization—have caused significant harm as well as important gains. How could the city monitor whether it was doing the right thing for its mentally ill citizens? How could it reduce the risk that a well-intentioned change would lead to degraded services for an already disadvantaged population?

One of the most common public reactions to managed care is a sense of confusion and powerlessness, often leading to distrust and anger. Medical journals, print media, late-night television, and movies paint portraits of anonymous insurance actuaries, backed by powerful and venal managed care executives, who thwart the needs of the sick by erecting administrative barriers and by wielding secret criteria to deny care. There have been widespread calls to solve this problem by greater consumer empowerment. But what do the words in this slogan really mean? What is implied by the distinction between *patient* and *consumer*? What exactly is an *empowered* health care consumer? And, how can empowered consumers actually exert a meaningful influence?

Although questions about empowerment in the relationship between consumers and health care organizations are new, concerns about the balance of power in the relationship between patients and their physicians have been at the center of medical ethics since the 1950s (Faden and Beauchamp, 1986). Before World War II, the dominant model for the patient–doctor relationship was paternalism. Paternalistic physicians used their knowledge, skill, and presumably benevolent attitudes to decide what was right for their patients. The phrases "doctor's orders" and "doctor knows best" were used with a straight face and without quotation marks. Since the 1950s, however, attitudes towards paternalism have undergone a sea change. Under the banner of *informed consent* we have seen a steady evolution toward new forms of patient–physician relationship, founded on respect for the *autonomy* of the patient.

In the new autonomy-respecting models of professional ethics, physicians foster trust and show regard for their patients by providing the information patients need, helping them clarify their preferences and values, and collaborating with them to develop and monitor the treatment plan (Emanuel and Emanuel, 1992). As we described in the previous chapter, health-care organizations should be expected to build a similar relationship with their consumer/members. In relation to the organizations through which they receive their care, consumers want to be informed about decisions and policies in an understandable manner and to influence the decisions and policies that touch on their interests and values. Central areas of concern include the benefit package, processes for interpreting benefits, medical necessity criteria, and the breadth of the provider network. Respect for autonomy in the realm of the patient–doctor relationship corresponds directly to empowerment in these areas of the consumer–health-care organization relationship.

In the broadest sense, the quest for consumer empowerment expresses the fundamental moral insight of democracy. Individuals should have maximum feasible opportunity to make their own choices and shape their own destinies. For patients with their physicians, maximum feasible opportunity means robust informed consent. For consumers with their health plans, maximum feasible opportunity means *empowerment*—being able to participate in shaping the policies and practices of the plan. Health care is a fundamental good, and health plans are the vehicle U.S. society currently uses to allocate that good. Democratic values require maximum opportunity for individuals to influence the processes through which health care is allocated. In practical terms, health organizations cannot expect to be able to implement policies that inevitably entail disappointment without grass roots support from within the population they serve, any more than democratic governments can do their work without the consent of the governed (Emanuel, 1991).

Albert Hirschman's classic book *Exit, Voice, and Loyalty* provides a key framework for thinking about the different dimensions of consumer empowerment in the American managed care system (Hirschman, 1970). From his perspective as an economist, Hirschman identified *exit* and *voice* as the basic strategies for influencing the performance of economic enterprises such as insurers and other health care organizations. In the insurance context, *exit* means disenrollment from one health plan and purchase of a new one; *voice* refers to the range of ways consumers can influence the enterprise without leaving it.

The theory behind America's system of competing insurance plans largely depends on exit as the major source of consumer influence. Dissatisfied patients will take their business elsewhere. According to the dominant theory, consumers are empowered by being able to vote with their feet. However, as Marc Rodwin has argued, U.S. health-policy thinking has overemphasized exit and neglected voice as a key empowerment strategy (Rodwin, 1997). While the idea that consumer exit will discipline health-care organizations makes good theory, more than half of the U.S. population has no choice of health plans, and even those who do are reluctant to switch if it means giving up trusted clinicians. Patients generally discover their dissatisfaction with a health plan when they become ill and undergo treatment. However, once they have what in actuarial terms is called a *preexisting condition,* they may not be able to switch their care to another insurer without a delay in eligibility for treatment of the condition. These realities of the insurance process constrain the degree to which exit can realistically be the source of consumer power. Free market ideology and the realities of insurance diverge in a way that creates major problems for U.S. health-care policy.

The United States cannot have an ethically admirable managed care system unless—in Hirschman's terms—consumers are empowered with effective voice in addition to their opportunity to exit. Voice is an "upstream" organizational process that seeks to guide and shape an ongoing consumer–health plan relationship, in contrast to exit, which acts "downstream." Voice is negotiation. Exit is divorce. Processes that enhance the degree to which consumers can influence policy and practice create voice and foster empowerment.

In the next section we discuss two federal programs that pushed consumer participation into the political spotlight—Community Health Centers, launched in 1965, and Health System Agencies, intoduced in 1974—and important contributions to consumer empowerment made by the National Committee for Quality Assurance (NCQA). We then describe three exemplary organizational approaches to consumer empowerment: the *consumer governance* model at Group Health Cooperative, the *consumer participation* model in public sector mental health programs in Massachusetts and Philadelphia, and the newly emerging Internet-based models that seek to transform the individual into an empowered *consumer purchaser*.

BACKGROUND

In 1965, when President Lyndon Johnson's war on poverty revealed major health impairments among the poor, the Office of Economic Opportunity launched an ambitious initiative for development of Community Health Centers to serve medically deprived populations. The community activists and community-oriented clinicians who pioneered the movement envisioned a radical new form of community–clinician partnership that would put the community in control of its health services. Not surprisingly, when Richard Nixon (1968–1974) and Gerald Ford (1974–1976) replaced the Kennedy/Johnson administrations (1960–1968), the left-leaning Office of Economic Opportunity was disbanded. Community Health Centers, however, survived. Responsibility for them was transferred to the Public Health Service.

Although Community Health Centers currently serve more than 11 million low-income clients, and although there are upwards of a thousand centers distributed among all 50 states, the centers have had remarkably little influence on the course of U.S. health policy. In order to overcome opposition from organized medicine and to escape a near-death experience during the Reagan years (1980–1988), supporters of the centers narrowed their focus from community development to provision of medical services. Whereas the founders of the movement hoped the new centers would lead to overall national health reform, in order to sustain any program at all, it was necessary to define it clearly as medicine for the poor. Thus, although regulations require that consumers must be a majority of the governing board, there has been virtually no transmission of lessons regarding consumer empowerment to the rest of the health-care system. The governance experience at Community Health Centers has not been a factor in the public debate about the role of the consumer in health-care organizations.

Despite the fact that Community Health Centers maintain consumer-dominated boards, the ill-fated National Health Planning and Resources Development Act of 1974 has had a greater influence on the evolution of mainstream thinking regarding consumer participation. This law, crafted by the Nixon administration to address accelerating health-care costs, sought to control health-care inflation through the creation of 200 consumer-dominated regional planning bodies called Health Systems Agencies. In its 12-year life, the Health Systems Agency program was entirely ineffective in controlling costs. But because the Health Systems Agencies—unlike the Community Health Centers—were placed squarely at the interface of professional provider groups, hospitals, and insurers, they created significant health system waves.

As James Morone and Theodore Marmor have shown, the primary lesson about consumer empowerment from the experience of the Health Services Agencies is a negative one—what *not* to do (Morone and Marmor, 1983). The law, which specified in great detail how consumer representatives should be chosen, was based on the hope that the selection process would create a mirror of the community by mixing and matching consumer representatives in accord with community demography. The anticipation was that if the Health Systems Agencies were a simulacrum of the community, they would be seen as a legitimate source of priorities and limits. The legislation envisioned that if the agencies could mirror the makeup of their communities, they would be able to make bold, forceful decisions that would command acceptance. Instead, the law fostered an avalanche of litigation by groups who felt they were being left out. The agencies themselves had no statutory power, so the results of their deliberations had no bite.

In retrospect, however, the otherwise unsuccessful Health Systems Agencies contributed in a serendipitous manner to the potential for consumer empowerment in the future. From their inception in 1974 to their defunding in 1986, the Health Systems Agencies undermined the longstanding assumption that doctors and hospitals know best in the realm of health policy. Consumers came to the table as equals in the policy-planning process. Once the power equation had been altered in multiple settings across the country, there was no going back. One way or another, the consumer voice would henceforth insist on being heard in the domain of health system policy.

Within the current landscape of managed care in the United States, neither the ideals of consumer empowerment embodied by Community Health Centers nor the structure of consumer voice provided by the Health Systems Agencies has a clear descendant. There exist umbrella advocacy groups, such as Families USA, the American Association of Retired Persons (AARP), and Public Citizen, that represent core constituencies in major health policy debates at the national level. But the relationship between health-care organizations and individual consumers has received relatively little attention. One important exception to this vacuum has been the work of NCQA. First established by a consortium of major purchasers and insurers, NCQA functions as the primary vehicle of health plan accreditation in the United States. NCQA accreditation, awarded after intense scrutiny of documents and in-depth site visits, means that an organization has demonstrated a certain level of performance in many defined domains of organizational responsibility. Within these domains, NCQA has set standards that embody a vision of an appropriate consumer–health plan relationship. Meeting these standards does not assure ethical excellence, but the standards do establish minimal expectations that nearly all health plans in the United States recognize as important elements of consumer empowerment.[1]

The vision of consumer empowerment that emerges from NCQA standards centers on the member's right to information and the health-care organization's responsibility for providing that information. The first standard under "Members' Rights and Responsibilities" states, "Members have a right to receive information about the managed care organization, its services, its practitioners and providers and members' rights and responsibilities."[2] The standards require the organization to provide each member "with the information needed to understand benefit coverage and obtain care."[3] In the area of quality improvement (QI), however, members are only entitled to information if they ask for it: "Upon request, the managed care organization makes available to its members and practitioners information about its QI program. . . ."[4]

NCQA standards provide clear and consistent support for active consumer participation in the treatment planning process. This is stated as "a right to participate with practitioners in decision making regarding their health care"[5] and "a right to candid discussion of appropriate or medically necessary treatment options."[6] There is no expectation, however, that members will participate in developing, evaluating, and revising organizational policies and practices. Thus, while the organization is required to involve "appropriate, actively practicing practitioners in its development or adoption of [utilization management (UM)] criteria and in the development and review of procedures for applying the criteria,"[7] required member involvement is limited to an annual survey "regarding their satisfaction with the UM process"[8] and to receiving written notification of the reason for any denials of service.[9]

NCQA standards also set extensive requirements for regular assessment of member satisfaction with multiple aspects of organizational performance. The standards establish a four-phase process: assessment of satisfaction; analysis of the responses; implementation of improvement activities; and evaluation of the effectiveness of these interventions. Surprisingly, while the health-care organization is required to inform "practitioners and providers of the results of member satisfaction activities," there is no requirement that the members themselves must also be informed.

In the NCQA standards, member satisfaction surveys, complaints, and appeals are the vehicles for the expression of member voice. The language of the standards and their rationales clearly place a high value on member empowerment, but the mechanisms for promoting that empowerment are limited to providing information, and assessing satisfaction, and responding to complaints and appeals. A more active partnership in which members participate in shaping policies and practices is consistent with NCQA objectives but goes well beyond what NCQA standards currently require. The current NCQA standards are thus best seen as a starting point, not a finished achievement (Sabin et al., 2001).

ETHICAL VALUES AND CENTRAL ETHICAL OBLIGATIONS

It is easy to state the central ethical obligations for consumer empowerment in health care because they are the core ethical commitments of democracy itself. Individuals should have maximum feasible opportunity to make their own choices and shape their own destinies with regard to fundamental goods like health and health care. The challenge is not in stating the core value that underlies consumer empowerment, but in addressing two central ethical dilemmas with regard to implementing it.

First, the primary ethical challenge for health care organizations facing limited resources is deciding how to provide the best possible care for each individual patient and the insured population as a whole within a budget. This challenge involves setting priorities and making trade-offs. To date, however, the consumer role in health care has been most powerful in advocating for what in the political sphere are called special interests. Breast cancer patients fight for breast cancer services. AIDS advocates demand fast tracking of AIDS drugs. Families of the mentally ill lobby for psychiatric benefits. Grateful patients endow programs run by the doctors and hospitals that treated them.

Given this natural human penchant to focus on ourselves, our families, and the causes we have been touched by, health-care organizations and, more broadly, health policy leaders, have reason to fear that empowered consumers could make the already difficult challenge of setting priorities and making trade-offs even harder. They fear that, while managed care organizations must operate within the constraints of budgets and population needs, consumers will inevitably fight for more for themselves, regardless of competing interests. The natural role for the empowered consumer is to advocate for the cause he or she is committed to, not to focus on fair limits and equitable distribution of limited resources. The first ethical dilemma is, thus, how to integrate consumer empowerment with the organization's stewardship responsibilities.

The second dilemma involves the question of whether consumer empowerment and management itself are compatible. Many of the Community Health Center and Health Systems Agency efforts bogged down in local politics and consumer–professional strife. Support for consumer participation at the organizational level largely waned in the 1980s, except within the narrow confines of health centers for the poor. The apparent lesson that consumer participation leads to strife and organizational turmoil was not lost on the corporations that rose to lead the U.S. managed care system. Health-care organizations fear they will lose their ability to manage effectively in a demanding marketplace if consumer/members significantly increase their power. Consumer empowerment could compete with clinical effectiveness, managerial efficiency, and ultimately, financial integrity if member participation undermined an organization's focus and ability to make quick decisions.

The goal of consumer empowerment is for consumers to receive the information they need to understand how their health system works, the opportunity to make their preferences and concerns known, and the tools with which they can exert influence. To assess consumer empowerment, we examine the clarity and effectiveness with which the organization pursues each of these different components. Our list of central ethical obligations for exemplary performance in consumer empowerment is shown in Table 4–1.

Consumer Empowerment through Governance–Group Health Cooperative of Puget Sound

Group Health Cooperative is unique in the United States as a health organization that has actually been governed by consumers for more than 50 years. Group Health finds its origins in the consumer cooperative movement that began in nineteenth-century England, in which consumers organized and owned not-for-profit organizations that addressed shared needs, like buying and selling agricultural products.

As described in *To Serve the Greatest Number* (the history written to commemorate the cooperative's 50th anniversary in 1997), the original incorporators educated themselves about group medical practice and launched the cooperative by purchasing a medical group and hospital. Although the degree of consumer activism has ebbed and flowed, Group Health has remained a consumer-governed organization with an elected consumer board throughout its existence. And there should be no mistake—this is a board of directors with full governance authority, not just an advisory board.

In 1947 100% of Group Health Cooperative enrollees were formal members of the cooperative. There was no way of participating in the care program without belonging to the cooperative. With growth and structural change over Group Health Cooperative's 55-year history, this percentage of full membership in the cooperative has dropped, much as the percentage of the population that registers and votes in national elections has dropped. Currently only 40,000 of the approximately 600,000 enrollees are members of the cooperative, despite the elimination of the requirement for paying a fee to become a member. Allowing for enrollees who are under the ordinary voting age, approximately 10% of potentially eligible cooperative voters are registered as members. And of these 40,000 members, only

Table 4–1. Central ethical obligations for consumer empowerment

ETHICALLY EXEMPLARY ORGANIZATIONS MUST:

1. Ensure that members have ready access to understandable information about policies and practices.
2. Seek diligently to understand members' preferences with regard to their health care.
3. Allow members to exert influence on the content of decisions and policies.

approximately 15,000 exercise their rights of membership by voting regularly. From the perspective of consumer participation, the good news is that Group Health Co-operative has sustained a robust structure of consumer governance for 55 years. The bad news is that active participation in the governance process is at a relatively low level, compared to earlier periods of Group Health Cooperative history.

Candidates for the board of trustees are elected by mail ballot or by in-person voting at the annual membership meeting. In recent years the meeting has been conducted on Saturday at the University of Washington in Seattle. The meeting includes a health fair, a report on the state of the organization, an educational panel and discussion, voting on resolutions, and a report of election results. The meeting notice contains campaign statements from the candidates for the board of trustees. In 1999, seven candidates stood for four seats. Each was asked to answer two questions: "What are the two most significant challenges facing the Cooperative?" and "What competencies would you bring to the governing board that could help address the challenges you cite?" The responses were notably informed, attentive to member, community, and organizational concerns, and strongly aligned with Group Health Cooperative's purposes.

Group Health Cooperative's decision in 1999 to leave Clallam County, a rural county in western Washington with strong consumer roots and enduring histori-cal ties to the cooperative, is the basis of the first vignette at the start of this chap-ter. The actual Clallam County story demonstrates that a consumer-governed organization can make tough choices when necessary for organizational survival. In response to a $48 million loss in 1997 and a $20 million loss in 1998, the con-sumer board voted that the cooperative should pull out of 14 rural counties, in-cluding Clallam. Board chair Debbie Ward's "Board Report" in the July/August 1999 *Member News* presents the rationale for this decision to the membership:

> For Group Health's network care to succeed, two elements must be in place. First, community providers must agree with our philosophy of care and see us as a clinical partner, not as an insurance contractor. Second, we should have a large enough pres-ence in their practices for it to make clinical and financial sense for us and for them. In the counties we are leaving, we weren't meeting one or both of the criteria.
>
> Leaving these service areas, where we have many loyal members, was a difficult decision. This decision affects some 21,000 members, or about 3 percent of our total enrollment. We regret having to disappoint any of our consumers. But now our fu-ture is clearer than it has been in many years. Group Health is united by a systematic set of health-improvement strategies and a single philosophy of medical manage-ment. We work in our own facilities with our own staff—and we work with commu-nity partners who share our philosophy.

The Clallam members who felt most betrayed were part of the founding group of the cooperative. Prior to the final decision, they lobbied vigorously for the coop-erative to stay in Clallam County. At the 1999 annual membership meeting, Clallam County members of the North Olympic Peninsula chapter of the senior caucus filed a resolution asking the cooperative to reverse the decision. Although the resolution was voted down, the management devoted tremendous effort to finding alternative solutions to address the wishes of the small group of loyal, long-term Clallam County members. In remembering this painful part of the organization's history, Group Health's CEO, Cheryl Scott, noted, "It wasn't just about their providers or the health plan—it was about the organization they had helped to found. It was a very meaningful personal relationship to them." The Clallam County incident shows that a consumer-governed organization was prepared to make a tough decision to protect the commons, but at the same time was determined to conduct itself with heart by working so diligently to minimize the impact on their fellow consumers.[10]

Group Health Cooperative's form of consumer governance is an internationally recognized exemplary practice. The fact that it has existed for more than 55 years proves that consumer governance can work. The fact that it is so little emulated in other organizations in the United States, apart from the typically small, federally sponsored Community Health Centers, however, proves that it is a remarkable achievement, not readily duplicated. One large factor in its success is the local political climate. After World War II, Washington State was joked about as the "Soviet of Washington." The cooperative movement in the United States was strongest there, and Group Health took its start at a propitious moment, when the health system needed to be reconfigured for the post-war period.

Group Health Cooperative provides a crucial counterexample to the conventional wisdom that a consumer-led organization cannot handle tough trade-off decisions rapidly enough or with an adequate sense of *realpolitik* to survive in a competitive market. The Group Health member meetings and the cooperative's board of directors have provided for responsible stewardship of organizational resources.

Organizations that want to strengthen consumer voice in their governance can learn from Group Health that consumers can bring consumer values and insights to an organization while recognizing at the same time the need to keep the organization itself viable and healthy. Consumer governance in health care is a rare phenomenon, but Group Health Cooperative proves that, in the right circumstances, it is wholly compatible with organizational success. Consumer governance can work, and when it does, it can beautifully demonstrate one way to sustain democratic values in competitive markets.

But does the Group Health example have any merit for health-care organizations not founded upon a cooperative structure? Can other forms of nonprofit organizations adopt some of the elements of consumer governance? More pointedly, what about for-profit corporations? With their alternative governance structure consisting of an outside board of directors directly accountable to a diffuse group of shareholders, and with their key stakeholders including investment bankers and Wall Street analysts, for-profit health care companies may compete in the same marketplace as a consumer-governed organization like Group Health, but their corporate realities may feel completely different. For-profit organizations may feel intensely accountable to consumers through the operation of the market, but true consumer governance is a foreign concept. We must consider the possibility that the assumptions built into the very idea of consumer governance are simply antithetical to for-profit companies.

There is, however, one structural element of potential consumer governance shared by Group Health, other nonprofit organizations, and for-profit corporations: a board of directors. While consumer governance at Group Health is expressed at annual member meetings, its true day-to-day power is exercised through its board of directors, who, quite consciously, speak of deciding how much power they should delegate to executives and managers. Far different are the boards of directors of many other health-care organizations, whether for-profit or nonprofit. Boards of directors can be tame, passive, and led through their traces by executives who have little regard for their input. Membership on boards of directors can occur through various pathways not always immune to cronyism, thereby producing a striking similarity of outlook and a narrow range of potential criticism and innovation.

We believe that the example of Group Health suggests that a strong consumer presence on the board of directors of any health-care organization might not only create ethical value by empowering consumers but might simultaneously strengthen an organization's competitive position. Strong, active, committed, experienced— consumers can be found with these virtues to serve on the board of any health-care organization. And they can bring with them a diversity not easily created otherwise. Although a full consideration of the interpersonal dynamics of boards of directors is beyond the scope of our discussion here, we do believe that consumers have more to offer as board members for health-care organizations than is generally recognized. Translating the lesson of Group Health in this way may allow a broad range of health care organizations to benefit from a governance approach to consumer empowerment.

Consumer Empowerment through Participation—Public Sector Mental Health in Philadelphia and Massachusetts

In the course of a study of exemplary public sector mental health programs that was conducted in conjunction with the BEST project, the BEST team identified a second distinct and illuminating approach to consumer empowerment. If *governance* is the process for setting and overseeing broad strategies, *management* is the process for realizing those strategies in action. Because public programs are subject to expectations that include open process and citizen oversight through electoral, legislative, and regulatory mechanisms, the ethos of public programs has been strongly oriented toward consumer participation in management. And since mental health has been a major public responsibility since the nineteenth century, mental health programs have had to be particularly creative in finding ways for consumers and family members to participate in program oversight. Among public sector mental health programs, Philadelphia and Massachusetts are recognized as flagship examples. Conceptually, what Massachusetts and Philadelphia have done is very simple. Whereas Group Health Cooperative puts consumers at the center of *governance*, Philadelphia (Sabin and Daniels, 2002) and Massachusetts (Sabin and Daniels, 1999) have pioneered ways of having consumers participate in the *management* process.

Philadelphia. On December 7, 1987, Pennsylvania Governor Robert Casey announced the closing of Philadelphia State Hospital (Byberry) in the ringing moral terms that characterized the deinstitutionalization movement: "Today, we're taking action that is both strong and compassionate [to] ensure that Pennsylvanians with mental illness and mental retardation will no longer be left out, left behind or forgotten." By 1989 the deaths of two former patients and the attempted suicide of another prompted intensive review of the closure plan (Acker, 1990). As part of the review, Joseph Rogers, then president of a consumer organization called Project SHARE, led a team of consumers that went into Byberry to interview patients about their needs for community care. Rogers proposed that consumers could be trained to gather quality-relevant data from users of the care system after the closure. His hypothesis was that interviewers with their own experience of psychiatric illness and treatment would be better able to elicit valuable feedback from current users of care.

In retrospect, Rogers's proposal was the right idea at the right time. Estelle Richman, then director of Philadelphia's mental services and later the city's managing director, feared that "we might wake up finding that we had put money into the community without accountability." Richman was convinced that "the best way to assess your services is through hearing from consumers and families" (E.B. Richman, personal communication, September 12, 2001). Rogers's concept and Richman's conviction led to the formation of Philadelphia's Consumer Satisfaction Team, Inc. in 1990, when Byberry finally closed.

The program has grown steadily from a team of four and a yearly budget of $138,000 at its inception to its current level of approximately 30 employees and a budget of $2.8 million. Its growth has been dynamic, but its mission has been stable:[11]

- To promote the satisfaction of individual consumers and people in recovery with their behavioral health (mental health and substance abuse) services.
- To be a link between consumers and the government entities that fund these services (the Office of Mental Health, the Coordinating Office for Drug and Alcohol Abuse Programs, and Community Behavioral Health).

- To promote the accountability of funders and providers of services to the people who use and depend upon these services.
- To contribute to an effective and cooperative behavioral health system.

Experts on organizational quality improvement put consumers at the heart of the improvement process. Quality cannot be evaluated and enhanced in a significant way without rich consumer involvement. But how should health systems define quality? And how should consumer perspectives enter in? In all areas of health care, consumers appear to care most about the perspectives of people like themselves. They want to hear about the care experience throughout an episode of illness—not just about satisfaction with single visits or global satisfaction with a health plan, as is so common in typical surveys (Edgman-Levitan and Cleary, 1996). In accord with this perspective, the Philadelphia Consumer Satisfaction Team uses trained consumers and family members to talk with service users about what they like and dislike in their treatment and report on what they are told.

The organization sends two-person teams, generally composed of a consumer (a current or past user of public mental health services) and a family member (a person who "consumes" mental health services through their involvement with a mentally ill relative), to make unannounced visits to mental health and substance abuse treatment sites. Of the approximately 10,000 consumer interviews it conducted in 2001, 53% focused on adult mental health, 37% on substance abuse, and 10% on child and adolescent services.

The Consumer Satisfaction Team defines its role very carefully and does not wish its teams to be confused as advocates, case managers, or monitors of therapy.[13] Reports quote and summarize what consumers actually say, avoiding interpretation and judgment. The providers we interviewed described the reports as clear, constructive, and respectful. The reports are sent at the same time to the provider and purchaser. The Consumer Satisfaction Team meets at least monthly with leadership from Community Behavioral Health and the other components of the Philadelphia Behavioral Health system.

A key ethical question about consumer participation in programs like the Consumer Satisfaction Team is whether it promotes better health outcomes. From a practical perspective, Philadelphia has voted with its purse—the annual allocation contract with the Consumer Satisfaction Team has steadily increased, as has the scope of the site visits. The following brief vignettes give an admittedly anecdotal picture of the impact of the program:

- Consumer feedback about emergency services revealed dissatisfaction with the gap between mental health and substance abuse components and with the linkages between the emergency services and other treatment sites. The emergency system was redesigned with a strong emphasis on shaping it around what consumers wanted. The redesigned system is in its third year of operation and is generally regarded as a meaningful improvement.

- A provider agency was concerned about a deteriorating residential site, and consumer perspectives confirmed this concern. The residential program was moved to a new site, about which consumers were very positive. While the agency was aware of the site problem, the feedback confirmed their analysis and helped them bring about the beneficial change.

When asked about the impact of consumer feedback, Loretta Ferry, executive director of Consumer Satisfaction Team, Inc. commented, "When we started doing this in 1990 we heard from 90% of the people we interviewed that they were not respected. In all of our reports that was a need for improvement—'respect for the consumers who live here.' We never hear that complaint any more! That is my favorite example."

Massachusetts. In 1992 Massachusetts became the first state to "carve out" its Medicaid Mental Health program and contract to have it managed by a company specializing in mental health managed care. The state was not satisfied with the original vendor, and in 1996 it shifted the contract to the Massachusetts Behavioral Health Partnership (the Partnership), which is part of ValueOptions, a large, national, for-profit mental health management company.

Massachusetts, like Philadelphia, has applied an activist philosophy as a purchaser of Medicaid Mental Health Services. According to Bruce Bullen, the Medicaid commissioner who guided the contracting process, "The prudent purchaser is not a passive buyer who merely selects the best value from among the choices offered, [but one] who has a vision of what health care can—and should—be, and who . . . express[es that vision] in purchasing specifications and work[s] with contractors to meet them" (Bullen, 1998).

A 20-member Consumer Advisory Council provides the hub from which the many spokes of consumer participation in the Partnership radiate. Massachusetts has been a hotbed of citizen/consumer activism since the Boston Tea Party era, and there are robust grassroots organizations of consumers and family members in all areas of the state. This is important, because no matter how positive the state and the Partnership might be about involving consumers in the managed care process, without a pool of effective consumer activists to work with, it could not accomplish much.

Approximately 15 consumer members, joined by high-level representatives of Medicaid, the Department of Mental Health, and other key state agencies, meet monthly for two hours with staff from the Partnership. The meetings focus on a small number of potentially high-impact issues, such as clinical guidelines, quality monitoring, and performance standards. The council is chaired by consumers elected from within the group. A membership subcommittee identifies potential members, who are selected on the basis of interest in participation, potential or demonstrated effectiveness in participatory roles, and the needs of the council for geographical, ethnic, age, and gender diversity. Participants are paid a small stipend for meetings.

At one council meeting, the Partnership medical director presented the draft of a guideline for treatment of schizophrenia. Members criticized the guideline for what they saw as overreliance on medication. At the next meeting, the medical director brought in the evidentiary basis on which he based his belief that antipsychotic medications should play a major role in the recommendations. The discussion shifted from a polarized critique of medication to a broader focus on the importance of emphasizing rehabilitation activities, including peer support programs, as well. Over several years, the Partnership has worked closely with the Consumer Advisory Council to foster a wide array of peer-led and recovery-oriented programs.

Aware of Philadelphia's positive experience with its Consumer Satisfaction Team, the Partnership, in 1998, contracted with two consumer organizations to sponsor development of a Massachusetts version of the same program. In conducting its initial set of survey interviews, the Massachusetts Consumer Satisfaction Team learned that patients did not understand the rights they had under the state's patient rights legislation. (The consumer-evaluators had put questions about patient rights into the survey out of their own concern about making sure that patients were treated with respect.) On the basis of the survey findings, several hospitals began to publicize the role of the human rights officer and to make that person more available to patients. Follow-up, six months later, showed that these improvements were continuing.

To support its multiple links to consumers, the Partnership has designated a highly skilled, full-time staff member to act as liaison between the organization and the consumer community. This is a boundary-crossing, translational role. Consumers often do not understand the organization and how best to influence managerial process, and the liaison provides regular coaching. Organizational staff often do not understand consumer perspectives and how to relate most constructively with the consumer community. Here, too, the liaison provides regular coaching. From the consumer members, the liaison knows what areas are of highest concern to the consumer community, and from being an employee of the Partnership, the liaison knows what program areas are in most need of consumer feedback.

In both Philadelphia and Massachusetts, the public agency that purchases Medicaid mental health services is strongly committed to acting as an agent for the beneficiaries. The concept of democratic process asks public agencies to provide this kind of focus on the consumer. To be an effective, empowered agent requires close and continuing collaboration with consumers, just as being an effective, empowered clinician requires detailed knowledge of the patient's goals and reactions to the treatment. In their approach to consumer participation, Philadelphia and Massachusetts are simply doing what health systems in a democracy are supposed to be doing. They empower themselves to pursue their mission of public service by empowering service recipients.

If expectations were enough to produce realities, these flagship examples would be replicated in all 50 states. There are at least two additional factors at work in the two settings. Estelle Richman, Bruce Bullen, and their colleagues provided unusually strong endorsement of the ethical imperative for consumer participation and unusually creative managerial leadership to make it happen. And in both Philadelphia and Massachusetts, consumers and family members had a history of organized activism. Just as public leaders in Philadelphia and Massachusetts brought well-honed values and skills to the management process, so did the consumer and family communities.

Consumer Empowerment through Individual Choice— New Approaches Involving the Web

For the last two decades, the United States has turned to the system of managed care programs competing in the marketplace as its vehicle for addressing the clinical, ethical, and political challenges of distributing health care services and setting limits on their provision. This has been done with a minimum of public understanding of the task itself. Group Health Cooperative is very unusual in the degree to which it engages its members in struggling with difficult trade-off decisions. And Oregon has received worldwide attention for its explicit process for setting priorities and its clear acknowledgment of the ethical imperative for healthcare rationing. But these are exceptions to the more general national effort to pretend that limits are not necessary and that hard choices can be avoided.

The intense backlash against the very concept of managed care indicates that the body politic has either not recognized the need for limits and priorities or, if it does, has not accepted the legitimacy of large health-care organizations as custodians of the process. After all, if the public believes that hard choices are unnecessary in health care, the disappointments patients and physicians experience under managed care must mean that an ethical crime is being committed. The backlash has led insightful critics like James Robinson to declare "the end of managed care" (Robinson, 2001), by which he means giving up on the effort to have insurance companies set priorities and allocate resources for the insured population. But since limits are unavoidable and choices must be made, who will do what needs to be done?

As of the writing of this book, the leading prophecy by health system prognosticators is that, since Americans are demanding more individual choice and control in the domain of health care, consumers themselves are the likeliest source for setting priorities and limits (Academy for Health Services Research and Health Policy, 2001). This trend towards individual control should not be surprising.

During the Revolutionary era, Patrick Henry demanded liberty or death. New Hampshire automobile license plates counsel us to "live free or die." In response to the steadily rising tide of health-care consumerism in the United States, entrepreneurial organizations are using the Internet to create a cornucopia of start-up ventures designed to give individuals radically increased control of their health-care choices. In the jargon of the insurance industry, consumers are being offered the opportunity to create their own personal insurance "products," rather than having the choice made for them by their employer or by picking from a limited range of fully formed health-plan choices (Goldsmith, 2000).

We include the new Web-based approaches to consumer empowerment in this discussion of exemplary practices because of the clarity of their moral vision, not because of an established track record of implementation. While still in its infancy, the emerging model represents a fundamental shift of moral vision. Until recently, health insurance reinforced the perception that "no man is an island," albeit much less so than in universal coverage systems like Canada and England. Populations create insurance by pooling their resources to protect themselves against shared risk. The populations may be defined by employment ("I have my insurance through General Motors"), plan membership ("I belong to Group Health Cooperative"), demography ("Since I'm over 65, I have Medicare"), or other factors. But the common element is the potential for individuals to see themselves as part of a larger population that must deal with the task of resource allocation in a clinically informed, ethically justifiable, and politically acceptable manner.

In contrast, the common element in the new Internet-based insurance programs is the idea that individuals can operate in isolation to create their own package of benefits. The role of the employer/purchaser turns on its head. Instead of negotiating with insurance plans for the employee, the employer gives the employee a defined contribution of money to be used towards health coverage. At this point, the employee goes to the website of one of the new Internet-based organizations and walks through a set of choices to create what one such program calls a personalized healthcare system.[14] Under this program, individuals choose their own network of primary care physicians, specialists, hospitals, laboratories, and more. Each component comes with a price attached, confronting the consumer directly with the challenge of making trade-offs based on personal calculations of value. Consumers are given full power to choose the networks and services for which they want coverage and are at full financial risk for the degree to which the package varies from the defined contribution. If the cost is less, they can purchase additional services or roll the money over to the next year. If their choices cost more than the defined contribution, they must pay the difference. A safety net indemnity insurance "wrap" covers such things as treatment needed from a provider outside of the personalized panel and care outside of the local area.

This consumercentric design has two distinctive ethical strengths. First, by asking consumers to "use [your] healthcare dollars to choose how and what [you] are willing to pay for healthcare, based on [your] individual needs and values,"[15] the programs educate consumers about the reality of limits and the need to make choices and trade-offs. Second, they squarely empower individual consumers to make these choices in accord with their own values, reflected in statements like "No one should control your healthcare needs but you."[16]

The distinguishing ethical strengths of the new Internet-based model are clear: educating consumers about the need for trade-offs and empowering them to make the key choices. The equally distinctive ethical limitations emerge by comparing the concept embedded in a so-called personalized health system with the original concept of Group Health Cooperative of Puget Sound. In both, the consumer is in a governance role. At Group Health Cooperative, however, that governance is exercised as part of a community of members. Within a community like the membership of Group Health Cooperative, the issue of setting priorities and making trade-offs is a matter for community deliberation and decision making. That deliberation focuses naturally on the needs of the population alongside the needs of individuals. In contrast, there is no "community" in the new Internet-based programs; individuals need only deliberate about their own preferences. This represents the ultimate in empowerment of the individual *qua* individual, but it obscures any conception of the communitarian values of social insurance and contributes to further disintegration of the already highly fragmented U.S. health care system.

The concept of defined contribution and the new Internet-based products capitalize on employer interest in stabilizing or reducing their costs and employee interest in maximizing choice and control. Union leaders and consumer activists, however, fear that defined contribution is a Trojan Horse for reducing employer support for health care—a loss of benefits that workers have fought for since World War II. For employees with enough wealth to meet their health care needs and wishes beyond what the defined contribution they receive will purchase, the new approach frees them from the need to cooperate with others in making trade-off decisions. But for those who are less well-off, the defined contribution approach may create a Hobson's-choice situation in which the individual is "empowered" to select adequate health coverage while sacrificing other central values or protecting those values by "choosing" inadequate health coverage.

The impetus for defined contribution/consumer choice products comes from employers seeking to minimize their costs and well-off employees seeking to maximize their choices. Proponents have not yet confronted the problems that arise from desegregating the risk pool. It is rational for healthy individuals who anticipate few health needs to choose lower-cost insurance with limited benefits, high deductibles, or both. The inevitable result is that programs offering more comprehensive coverage will experience increased costs per member since healthier members will have migrated to other insurance offerings. Worse yet, the savings that would accrue to the 85% of the population (who—for reasons of rational self-interest—might choose lower-cost products with less coverage) could pull so much money out of the system that care for the sickest 15%, whose care consumes 80% of the health-care budget, would be unaffordable. Such a scenario could provide the final nail in the coffin for the history of pooled-risk private health insurance in the United States. A process that began with the abandonment of mandatory community rating in the insurance industry may culminate in the atomization of risk at the individual level. If this is to happen anywhere, it will happen in the United States. This new version of consumer empowerment will be at the heart of many experiments that will test the moral vision of health care as a social good.

LESSONS LEARNED

Health-care organizations that must manage care under resource constraints face a daunting challenge. In the United States, these organizations are required to find the elusive balance between fidelity to the needs of individual patients and stewardship of the collective resources of populations. And they must strike this balance while fighting for their economic survival in a competitive market. The political process gives them no succor; without formal sanction or any effort to educate the public about what needs to be done, the political process delegates to these organizations the responsibility to set priorities, make hard choices, and ration care. Unless consumers and providers can be enlisted in co-managing this process, the already intense backlash against the very mention of managed care will only increase even further.

Alliances, in which the triad of health-care organizations, empowered consumers, and quality-minded providers incorporates clinical understanding, consumer values, and financial realities into collaboratively managed programs, embody an ideal for population-based care. This is not simply a challenge for U.S. managed care. The same issues are being struggled with, for example, by Provincial Health Plans in the Canadian single-payer system and District Health Authorities in the U.K. National Heath Service. Our field studies provide three specific lessons about exemplary practice that can be applied and further developed in a wide range of health-care systems.

First, and most important—in the right circumstances, consumers are able to consider the collective interests of the insured population as well as their personal interests. Consumers sitting on the Group Health Cooperative Board of Directors or the Massachusetts Behavioral Health Partnership Consumer Advisory Council have acted as stewards for the insured population, not as atoms of individual self-interest. In these settings, consumers served as custodians of the commons rather than as advocates for themselves. Human nature does not preclude consumer cooperation in the health-care management process.

Second, we identified two well-established strategies for promoting consumer empowerment—consumer governance and consumer participation. The fact that the governance model, applied at the Group Health Cooperative since 1947, has been reproduced so rarely shows that it is not easily transportable. The cooperative governance approach in its entirety is probably more applicable in national cultures with strong solidarity values than in the highly individualistic milieu of the United States. But the fact that it has survived, evolved, and thrived in a competitive market over the course of 55 years proves that consumer governance is more than a naïve ideal. And, as we have discussed, the contribution of consumers to boards of directors is an element of consumer governance that is widely applicable to health-care organizations of varying structures and cultures.

The Philadelphia Consumer Satisfaction Team and the Massachusetts Behavioral Health Partnership provide examples of how consumer participation can contribute in substantial ways to the direction of a managed care program. Meaningful participation, however, does not simply happen by inviting consumers to attend meetings. Just as organizations provide orientation and training for new managers, they must do the same for consumers. Then, as the two programs show especially clearly, the organization must ensure that consumers participate at key points of high leverage in the management process.

Third, the Internet will rapidly bring forward much more individualized approaches to consumer empowerment. By what is called *disintermediation* in Internet jargon, individuals will be able to assume directly many of the management functions currently carried out by health insurers. For individuals with the skill and resources to seize these new opportunities, the new technologies will be highly empowering. They carry the risk, however, of increasing inequality between relatively affluent, Internet-savvy consumers and less well-to-do, less Internet-literate members of the population. And, by moving the healthier members of risk pools to less-costly, less-comprehensive packages, the new products could reduce access for those with greater health care needs by driving up the cost of the products their interests lead them to choose.

Programs that set limits on health care can achieve legitimacy in the eyes of members and concerned stakeholders only if they are held accountable for the reasonableness of their limit-setting policies (Daniels and Sabin, 2002). Reasonable policies are those that seek an optimal balance between the needs of individuals and those of the population. Fair-minded people may disagree about how best to balance the needs of individual patients and the totality of an insured population. But any health care system that pools funds to provide care for individuals as part of an insured population must seek that balance if it hopes to be seen as legitimate.

Deliberating and deciding about how to balance individual and population values cannot be left to even the most expert and benevolent clinicians and managers. Setting health care limits fairly requires clinical knowledge and managerial expertise, but the ultimate choices must inevitably reflect values choices as well as knowledge and expertise. These ethical choices must ultimately be made in accord with consumer values.

All of the programs we studied shared this perspective, but they varied widely in the degree to which they actually involved consumers and consumer values in the management process. In order to overcome the impediment posed by the fear that a strengthened consumer role will reduce an organization's ability to weigh collective as well as individual interests and conduct itself with managerial efficiency, additional pro-consumer forces must be present.

For Group Health Cooperative, the conviction held by the early incorporators of the cooperative provided that impetus. In the "soviet of Washington" those convictions were held with unusual strength. The governance model embodies an ideal, but even in Washington State, it has been difficult to sustain the original cooperative vision.

In public sector programs the expectations of democratic process itself provide an additional driver, but the fact that programs like Philadelphia and Massachusetts are flagships shows that democratic expectations alone are not enough to ensure robust consumer empowerment. Distinctively committed leadership and a strong consumer community are also required.

The current surge of enthusiasm for the Internet-based model of direct consumer choice reflects a tentative marketplace conclusion that consumer-governance and consumer-participation approaches are not up to the task of setting limits in a politically effective manner. Although our observations in Massachusetts, Philadelphia, and Washington State suggest that consumers, empowered by governance or participation, can promote the collective enterprise of setting limits fairly, it appears that the U.S. system is heading toward a period of experimentation with much more individualistic mechanisms.

NOTES

1. The excerpts in the following section are from NCQA's Standards for the Accreditation of Managed Care Organizations (Effective July 1, 2001) and are available from NCQA or on the Web at <www.ncqa.org>.

2. Ibid. Rights and Responsibilities (RR) 1.1.

3. Ibid. Rights and Responsibilities (RR) 4.1.

4. Ibid. Quality Improvement (QI) 2.4.

5. Ibid. Rights and Responsibilities (RR) 1.3.

6. Ibid. Rights and Responsibilities (RR) 1.4.

7. Ibid. Utilization Management (UM) 2.2.

8. Ibid. Utilization Management (UM) 10.1.

9. Ibid. Utilization Management (UM) 6.2.

10. The Clallam County story came to a happy ending when an act of the legislature changed insurance regulations to allow individuals in the county to keep their coverage if they wished. The happy ending reflected the advocacy skills and tenacity of the Clallam County Cooperative members.

11. Information is available at <http://www.thecst.com>.

12. Information is available at <http://www.phila-bhs.org>.

13. The Consumer Satisfaction Team, Inc. (2000). *Annual Report: 2000*. Available from The Consumer Satisfaction Team, Inc., 520 North Delaware Avenue (7th floor), Philadelphia, PA 19123.

14. Information is available at <http://www.vivius.com>.

15. Information is available at <http//www.vivius.com/AboutUsMission Statement>.

16. Information is available at <http://www.vivius.com/aboutus>.

5

MEDICAL NECESSITY, COVERAGE DECISIONS, AND MEDICAL POLICY

Ronald Barnes is a 12-year-old boy who was born with a severely deformed left ear. As a young child, Ronald had reconstructive surgery on the ear that produced a satisfactory functional result, but the ear remained quite small and misshapen. As Ronald grew older, he was frequently teased by his schoolmates, and he suffered poor school performance as a result. As he neared adolescence, the impact on his life of his "ugly" ear escalated. In an attempt to alleviate mounting psychological problems, and with the recommendation of their pediatrician, Ronald's parents took him to see Dr. Schmidt, a plastic surgeon. Dr. Schmidt told them that, through new surgical techniques, she could restore the ear to a nearly normal appearance. Ronald and his family were ecstatic, and Dr. Schmidt requested preauthorization for the revision from the family's HMO, Ultima Care. Two weeks later the Barnes family received a brief letter from Ultima Care saying that coverage for treatment would be denied because it was a cosmetic procedure and therefore not "medically necessary." Confused and angry, Ronald's parents didn't know what they should do next.

Dr. Steven Bernstein is the senior medical director for Ultima Care HMO, based in Massachusetts. One morning Dr. Bernstein received a call about a 20-year old man, Henry Larson, an Ultima member, who had been hospitalized for a month after a serious car accident left him quadriplegic. As the time approached when he was to be moved from the hospital to a nearby rehabilitation facility, the patient's sister had called to request a benefit exception that would cover a transfer of Henry's care to the Shepherd Rehabilitation Center in Atlanta, Georgia, the rehabilitation center where the well-known actor Christopher Reeve received care after his injury.

The secretary soon had the patient's sister on the line. Dr. Bernstein began by expressing his sorrow at what had happened to her brother. Then he asked her to explain why she had asked for Henry's transfer to the Shepherd Center in Atlanta. Expecting to hear overly optimistic statistics and glowing testimony concerning the Shepherd Center's excellence, Dr. Bernstein silently prepared his counterargument: the local rehabilitation facility was excellent, and the patient's HMO insurance contract quite clearly restricted care to the HMO's local network. But something happened instead. The patient's sister never even mentioned the Shepherd Center. She explained that she was the oldest child in a family of seven; Henry was her youngest brother, and when their parents died young, she had raised him from the age of three. She was the only one in the family who could spend the time and effort to help Henry, to work with him daily, to encourage him, and to care for him. She wanted to maximize Henry's potential rehabilitation and get him home to continue this work as soon as possible. But she lived in Atlanta with her husband and two children.

As Dr. Bernstein listened to the personal details of the situation, he felt his initial resistance to the idea of the outside referral melt away. A transfer to the Shepherd Center in Atlanta was really the only way for Henry to receive the active support of his sister, whose role would be critical in maximizing Henry's recovery and in getting him out of a rehabilitation facility and back home quickly. Dr. Bernstein gave his OK to the request and subsequently aided in making sure that all necessary hospital records and clinical information were sent to Atlanta.

The patient's sister called back one month after Henry had been transferred to Atlanta. Henry was now living at home with her and, through intensive outpatient rehabilitation sessions, had stunned everyone by being able to take a few steps.

Jekyll and Hyde? Can Ultima Care really occupy both ends of the spectrum? In one case it uses a form letter to deny coverage, fulfilling the stereotype of the heartless, bean-counting HMO. In the second vignette, Ultima Care exercises a level of personal attention and patient advocacy that seems to rise above a bottom-line mentality to realize the best conceptions of coordinated care. How could Ultima Care's approaches and results seem so contradictory? Those experienced in the nuts and bolts of medical necessity decisions will understand. The purpose of this chapter is to make explicit the reason that health-care organizations that manage care and costs in a competitive system can find themselves twisted into knots over coverage decisions such as these. We will explore the complex interplay between scientific evidence and insurance language, between fidelity to the needs of the individual and commitment to the stewardship of population-based resources, and between organizational systems built to provide consistency and systems meant to identify exceptions to every rule. As an example of practical organizational ethics in health care, few tasks can match the political and ethical challenges of determining medical necessity.

That questions about medical necessity are so central to debates about managed care in the United States should come as no surprise. "Although we may list a specific service as a benefit, we will not cover it unless we determine it is medically necessary to prevent, diagnose, or treat your illness, disease, injury, or condition." So reads the contract language of a Blue Cross Blue Shield Service Benefit

Plan for federal employees. Similar language can be found in virtually every health insurance contract in the United States. The rapid introduction of new drugs, devices, and procedures means that any specific list of services covered for reimbursement would rapidly become obsolete, so insurance contracts have relied on broad language about the scope of coverage. It is into this semantic space that the term *medically necessary* has been inserted. Broad, bland, tantalizingly yet misleadingly inclusive, the concept of medical necessity seems a Rorschach blot into which any stakeholder in the health-care system can find what he or she is looking for. Physicians, of course, have traditionally believed that they hold the prerogative to make the medical decisions about which treatments and services are needed by their patients. Patients, increasingly well-informed about treatment options, have come to expect the freedom to seek out physicians who will work with them to provide the care they want.

But U.S. managed care organizations feel that they must be the masters of medical necessity. It is they, after all, who must master a Gordian knot, with one strand composed of duties to providers and patients, and another arising from duties to purchasers, to whom the managed care organizations are contractually responsible for the quality and cost of medical services. And so, who owns medical necessity? The ongoing struggle over the power to decide what care is given and paid for lies at the heart of the high emotion and intense regulatory, legislative, and legal efforts to define the role of managed care in the United States.

The issues and controversies surrounding the determination of medical necessity are in no way isolated to the fractious world of American managed care. In one way or another, every developed nation has its own versions of Ronald Barnes, the boy with the deformed ear, and his attentive, anxious parents and physicians. There are health administrators and medical directors in every country who confront cases like that of the paralyzed young man and his costly recovery. Every developed nation must wrestle with broad definitions of covered services and must consider how the boundaries of covered services should reflect available resources. They must also face the traumatic cases in which last or best hopes for individual patients fall outside those boundaries. The political and ethical legitimacy of decisions of medical necessity thus forms a fragile cornerstone of the health-care system of every developed nation.

BACKGROUND

The history of insurance coverage language is important for an understanding of the options available to organizations seeking exemplary practice in medical necessity determination and corresponding coverage decisions.[1] Modern health insurance programs in the United States began to take root following World War II.

Created largely by the hospital industry and medical professional organizations, these programs had two goals in mind: to help individuals spread the financial risks of medical problems and to ensure that physicians got paid. The only limitations in contract language were in their listing of the broad categories of covered services, and insurance companies routinely paid any claim made within those categories. Physicians' medical opinions during this time largely dictated coverage and were rarely challenged by insurers.

The omnipotence of physicians started to erode in the early 1960s when insurers began to pay more attention to questionable requests for payment, such as for hospitalization to administer weight-loss programs or to convalesce after a fall (Eddy, 1996). Financial competition among insurers had increased by this time, and with looser allegiance to the hospital and physician community, insurers had greater freedom to doubt the gospel that the judgment of physicians was an infallible guide to appropriate care. At first, insurers began to deny payment for only the most egregious cases. But if challenged in court, these denials were usually overturned by judges, who cited the lack of any contractual terms justifying the withholding of payment.

In response to these adverse legal decisions, insurers began to add clauses to their contracts that limited coverage to services that were *medically necessary* or *medically appropriate*. These terms were not always defined further, and even when they were, the definitions were limited to vacuous statements about services that were known to be effective and needed for the proper care of a condition. Left unspecified were the who and the what: Who exactly would determine whether a service was medically necessary, and what would be considered valid criteria for making the decision? Although these additions to contracts helped clarify the purpose and intended limits of coverage, they did not prevent insurers from losing in court. The courts' reasoning appeared to be that, although it was appropriate for an insurer to limit coverage based on medical necessity, a physician's decision to use a treatment was still considered to be de facto evidence of necessity—even in some cases where the treatments were outlawed in the United States (Hall and Anderson, 1992; Eddy, 1996).

It was not until the end of the 1970s that insurers responded by specifying in their contract language that medical necessity would be determined by the insurers themselves. Most contracts also stated that medical necessity explicitly excluded treatments that were experimental or investigational. During this decade, two further developments arose that would have far-reaching effects on attitudes toward medical necessity. The first of these was the appearance of academic work describing wide variations in the rates of certain surgical procedures across the United States (Wennberg and Gittelsohn, 1973). Rates of surgery for conditions such as hysterectomy varied more than ten-fold across defined geographic areas, without apparent justification. Both public and private purchasers of health care had to wonder whether, in some regions of the country, they were paying for a lot of unnecessary, and even inappropriate care. To address this question, the RAND Corporation initiated a series of studies on the appropriateness of various medical and surgical procedures in the mid-1980s. Their methods involved the convening of expert panels to produce specific clinical criteria that could be used to judge the appropriateness of a medical treatment or procedure. Applying these appropriateness criteria to the varying rates of procedures seen across the country, the RAND studies confirmed the worst fears of many: high levels of inappropriate care were being delivered (Chassin et al., 1987). Not only did these findings spur purchasers and insurers to seek new control over medical decisions, but this academic approach challenged the very basis for determining what was clinically appropriate. While individual physicians could still make the first judgment of what was appropriate for their patients, the ultimate standard was no longer to be the local medical community but rather a mixture of scientific evidence and national consensus opinion that could be used by the insurer to make an ultimate determination.

The second major development of the 1970s to affect attitudes toward the idea of medical necessity was the growing awareness among large private purchasers of health insurance that the skyrocketing cost of health care premiums was seriously eroding their competitive position in the global marketplace. The large automakers were prominent in coming to realize the economic drag of their health-care obligations in comparison to the lower costs born by competitors in other countries. Automakers made public calculations showing that the cost of health insurance made up a higher proportion of the total cost of a new automobile than the steel needed to build it. When combined with the growing knowledge of the wide variation in the provision of health care services and the understanding that many surgical and medical treatments appeared to be inappropriate, this clarification of the economic burden of health care costs provided an irresistible force leading many purchasers to join a rush into managed care.

And yet, throughout the 1980s and even the 1990s, while managed care became the predominant form of insurance coverage in the country, and as for-profit insurers came to dominate the landscape, the definition of medical necessity in insurance language evolved very little. Partly because of professional resistance to the implications of the RAND study and partly because of the cost and technical difficulty of assessing the appropriateness of hundreds of procedures, many insurance definitions of medical necessity remained vague, without any inclusion of the concepts of appropriateness or cost-effectiveness. During the planning phase of the Clinton administration's effort to reform national health care, a taskforce was given the job of creating an expanded definition of medical necessity. This effort, perhaps the best chance in the last decade for a clarified definition of the term, died along with Clinton's other proposals for national health care reform in 1994 (Bergthold, 1995).

THE CURRENT LANDSCAPE AND KEY ISSUES

Unresolved issues of the definition and application of medical necessity continue to plague the U.S. health-care system. In the 1990s, as public and professional concern coalesced into a backlash against managed care, some medical necessity controversies were erased, at least temporarily, by state legal mandates. Prominent among such measures, now widespread, were those that recognized coverage for emergency services based on the so-called prudent layperson standard of medical necessity. During the mid-1990s, there was also a flourish of state legislation to guarantee coverage for services that some health insurers had not universally considered medically necessary. These services included specific medical treatments, such as bone marrow transplant for advanced breast cancer or reconstructive surgery following mastectomy. Legislation also guaranteed coverage for certain locations and durations of care, such as the publicly popular guarantee of a minimum of two days' hospital stay following normal vaginal delivery.

But the idea of adding further unique services to a growing list of state mandates soon lost its appeal as lawmakers and others realized that rapid changes in scientific knowledge and technology made state legislation an awkward and imprecise method for managing health care. Instead, adverse determinations of medical necessity, commonly known as denials, came into the spotlight. Soon the focus of debate about medical necessity had shifted largely to the rights of patients to have a timely and fair external review of coverage denials. In a May 2000 policy report on external review programs, researchers for the Kaiser Family Foundation found that the number of state external review programs had grown to include 32 states and the District of Columbia (Kaiser Family Foundation, 2000). In addition, many private health plans (including Aetna US Healthcare, United Healthcare, Health Net, PacifiCare Health Systems, the California Association of Health Plans, and ultimately, the American Association of Health Plans) had announced that their organizations would voluntarily provide enrollees access to external review when coverage was initially denied. Further, the National Committee on Quality Assurance (NCQA), a private body that accredits HMOs, expanded its accreditation standards to require plans to make available external review of medical necessity denials, effective in July 2000.

External review programs, however, did not prove immune from concerns about their scope and fairness. Some external review programs explicitly exclude disputes over benefit/coverage limitations in the health insurance contract and restrict their focus to disputes over medical necessity or other clinical judgments. But the distinction between medical necessity and other types of coverage disputes can lie in the eye of the beholder, and some policy analysts have worried that any restriction on external review may give an insurer the opportunity to set up various levels of protection for different kinds of denials (Kaiser Family Foundation, 2002).

Even when disputes do reach an external review program, there can be great variation in the way the review is handled. Most state and voluntary external review programs depend on organizations known as Independent Review Organizations (IROs). Accreditation and standardization across IROs are in their infancy. State regulations have also introduced variation into IRO decisions. At least six states define in law or regulation a standard for medical necessity that external reviewers should follow in evaluating cases. The individual reviewer's or IRO's definition of medical necessity is substituted for that of the plan in at least 14 states, whereas under at least eight state laws and many voluntary programs, IROs and their reviewers must make decisions based on the managed care plan's definition of medical necessity. This variability in the rules for IRO decisions, along with continuing concerns about barriers to consumer access and potential conflicts of interest for IROs that do other business with the health plans, have tarnished the once bright hope that external review programs, by themselves, would provide a universal safety valve for all medical necessity problems.

And so, despite the early wave of state-legislated mandates covering certain health care services and after the spread of external review programs, serious debates continue to rage over the internal handling of medical necessity determinations by health plans. Preauthorization for tests and treatments, one of the methods through which health plans have controlled medical necessity determinations, continues to be a lightning rod for discontent. There is perhaps no more enduring image of the managed care approach to medical necessity than that of the faceless bureaucrat, the bean counter, who sits in ignorant and venal judgment upon the needs of patients and the decisions of dedicated physicians. The fact that state and NCQA standards require that only licensed physicians make the "no" decisions for coverage denials has not penetrated the consciousness of the public, nor placated the ire of practicing physicians.

Practicing physicians continue to show significant anger and distrust toward what they view as onerous requirements for preauthorization. Largely because of this ongoing negative impression on the part of physicians and the public, UnitedHealthcare announced in 1999 that it would become the first major national health plan to eliminate prior authorizations for most tests, procedures, and admissions. UnitedHealthcare's move was interpreted by many as a promise to hand back to physicians the power to determine what was medically necessary for individual patients. The event was hailed as a turning point in the evolution of managed care. But within months, many physicians were complaining that the insurer was still in charge through the use of tight formularies, restricted specialist networks, and the hidden threat of deselection for those physicians who used too many expensive services (Terry, 2000). Within the community of health plans, few have followed UnitedHealthcare's lead. Although many insurers have cut back on the scope of preauthorization, nearly all retain some elements, and none has ceded a significant part of its authority to make decisions about medical necessity.

On other fronts, similar battles continue to rage. An April 2000 agreement on medical necessity determination between Aetna US Healthcare and the Texas Attorney General's office was initially touted as including important protections for patients and physicians, but the American Medical Association (AMA) lost little time in heaping condemnation upon the agreement for leaving medical necessity determination in the hands of Aetna and not specifying the role of the treating physician. The head of the AMA wrote to the Texas Attorney General, "The [settlement's] definition of 'medical necessity' is very close to Aetna's contractual definition, which allows Aetna to override the decision of a treating physician and inappropriately considers costs in a clinical context" (Klein, 2000). A spokesman for Aetna responded that "there's no question that Aetna, as a health plan, has that ultimate responsibility, and if physician groups are suggesting otherwise, that would be a pretty radical change" (Klein, 2000).

But if health plans are responsible for medical necessity determinations, what little is known about the process through which they make these determinations is not encouraging. In 1999 the Stanford University Center for Health Policy led a research project to learn about how medical necessity decisions were being made by health plans and provider groups in California. They found striking variation in all elements of the process, with evidence that these variations were causing problems for consumers and providers alike. In one of the hypothetical cases used in the research, investigators reviewed three plan coverage guidelines for a single condition and found only two areas of agreement among over a dozen factors studied. When these medical directors were asked whether they would approve or deny the hypothetical treatment, all three had different responses, and two responses contradicted their own plan's or group's coverage guidelines.

In summary, in an age of cost control, the lack of consensus on medical necessity continues to haunt those who are responsible for constructing an ethically transparent and legitimate system for the allocation of limited health-care resources. Physicians, patients, and the public at large have had little reason to trust that large, often for-profit, corporations will make medical necessity determinations fairly. And what little evidence there is suggests that health plans and provider groups, in fact, do not have reliable, transparent systems for making these decisions. Medical policy has failed to be reliable. It has failed as a means of public understanding of how health plans make hard choices. Instead, medical policy has been a black box, often a proprietary black box, kept explicitly hidden away from physicians and patients. But the tide has turned in recent years, and now many health plans are aware that medical necessity determinations frame the public face of managed care. The time is ripe for the identification and sharing of exemplary approaches to the quandary of medical necessity.

ETHICAL VALUES AND CENTRAL ETHICAL OBLIGATIONS

Medical directors and organizations do not see the process of determining medical necessity as standing alone; rather, it exists embedded within the broader framework of medical policy. Medical policy, in a sense, is the organization's procedural attempt to answer the riddle of medical necessity. Medical policy is created by complex and overlapping steps through which each organization designs benefit coverage plans; determines which treatments and other services are effective and appropriate; makes the decisions of when to change, bend, or break existing coverage policies; and adjudicates disputes over these decisions. The common labels given to these components of medical policy are (*1*) benefit design; (*2*) technology assessment; (*3*) coverage decision making; and (*4*) benefit adjudication (see Figure 5–1).

The core ethical dilemmas in the domain of medical necessity arise out of the fundamental conflict between, on one hand, the value of physician and patient autonomy to decide what is medically beneficial for an individual patient, and on the other, the duty of the health plan (or capitated provider group, or district, or province) for stewardship over quality and costs. Compassion lines up on the side

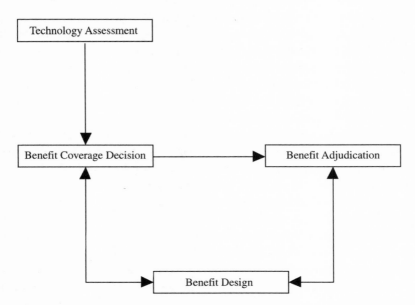

Figure 5–1. Medical necessity: the making of medical policy. The process of making medical policy consists of several different components that feed into each other and interact in often complex ways. The key elements in this chain are: (*1*) Technology Assessment; (*2*) Benefit Coverage Decision; (*3*) Benefit Design; and (*4*) Benefit Adjudication.

of recognizing the individual's special needs; fairness and prudence take their place in support of a hard-nosed approach and the ultimate justice of saying "no." This ethical tension is itself surrounded by another organizational value: every health-care organization wishes to survive and prosper. The value of organizational financial success in competitive markets thus accentuates and brings close to home the potential tension between care and costs.

The various components of the so-called medical policy machine are the tools with which a health plan strikes a balance between its competing values. In so doing, each health plan must make decisions about the allocation of resources that seek to balance the needs and desires of purchasers, the entire population of enrolled members, and individual patients. Each health plan in the United States must make decisions about how to define and determine medical necessity while competing for survival and growth in a fiercely competitive market environment. As it makes these decisions, each health plan expresses its own culture and values through the way it identifies and uses scientific data, includes or excludes the values of multiple stakeholders, and manages disputes arising over specific coverage decisions.

As we have argued earlier, for any set of decisions that must manage conflicting ethical values, a pragmatic analysis of normative obligations will focus primarily on the decision-making process and not on the specific decisions themselves. Thus the emphasis in our ethical analysis in the domain of medical necessity is not on the *right decision* but primarily on the *right methods* for making decisions. There is, however, even within this procedural focus, an additional part of ethical thinking that recognizes the importance of the character and virtues of the decision maker or the decision-making organization. In that vein, Table 5–1 summarizes the central ethical obligations for any health-care organization responsible for determining medical necessity and rendering coverage decisions as part of its broader medical policy. There are procedural requirements; there are also normative obligations of intent, character, and long-term goals. These obligations dovetail with those presented earlier in our chapter on organizational ethics. When taken together, these obligations represent the specific elements of a medical policy process that can make strong claims for ethical legitimacy. The deeper foundation from which springs a requirement for these specific elements is our argument that medical policy, in order to be ethical, must embody the following broad components of fairness and justice: (*1*) accessibility, (*2*) scientific rationality, (*3*) consistency, (*4*) transparency to outside observers, and (*5*) a caring and humane character. These are the core ethical virtues of any exemplary medical policy program out of which emerge determinations of medical necessity.

Benefit Design

One of the central ethical obligations of benefit design is to assure a minimum acceptable level of health-care coverage for all enrollees. We heard several organizations tell stories of how the marketplace and/or purchasers were pushing to have

Table 5-1. Central ethical obligations for medical necessity, coverage decisions, and medical policy

Benefit Design

1. Involve reasonable mechanisms to ensure a minimum acceptable level of health-care coverage for all enrollees.
2. Underwrite benefit packages sufficiently to support a long-term commitment to patients, purchasers, and physicians.
3. Include provisions to protect those patients at greatest risk when making changes in benefits that reduce coverage or limit therapeutic options.
4. Provide potential enrollees and current members with information on benefit structure, exclusions, and limits to support their informed selection of health plans and their options for health care, once enrolled.
5. Minimize financial conflict of interest for the designers and marketers of benefit packages.

Technology Assessment

1. Ensure that appropriate scientific and clinical expertise is available for all assessments.
2. Minimize financial conflict of interest for all participants in technology assessments.
3. Use a standardized and explicit process to judge the effectiveness of a medical service.
4. Clearly define the roles of those individuals involved in technology assessment and those involved in coverage decisions.

Coverage Decisions

1. Seek out and include appropriate clinical expertise.
2. Base coverage decisions in scientific evidence, with the evidence and rationale made available publicly to both patients and physicians.
3. Acknowledge and disclose fully the inclusion of cost considerations in decision making.
4. Ensure that coverage decisions are not linked in any way to direct financial rewards and/or performance evaluations of decision makers.
5. Provide timely access to senior medical personnel for physicians and patients who differ with an initial coverage decision.

Benefit Adjudication

1. Ensure that treating physicians have ready access to organizational channels through which to seek needed care for their patients that may extend beyond benefit limits.
2. Communicate clearly the entire process for benefit adjudication to members in enrollment information and to patients initiating the process.
3. Create a time-sensitive process.
4. Make available appropriate clinical expertise for the review of all decisions.
5. Seek out and consider multiple perspectives, including those of treating physicians and patients.
6. Place great value on consistency (treating like cases similarly), yet explicitly provide flexibility for exceptional cases.
7. Provide patients with a clear and ready recourse to an independent review of their cases by a qualified external review body that is entirely free of conflict of interest.
8. Perform internal review of adjudication decisions to seek continual improvements in quality, consistency, and integration with other organizational processes (e.g., benefit design).

important pieces of health-care benefits, such as organ transplantation, "stripped out" of benefit packages in order to create lower-priced offerings. Other health plans saw the first signs in their markets of a trend toward higher deductible and co-payment benefit packages. Purchasers were simply not going to be able to keep pace with health-care premiums slated to rise 20% or more for several consecutive years. They wanted to empower their employees by giving them greater choice among benefit packages with disparate levels of deductibles and co-payments. The impetus for this change was clear: purchasers hoped to be able to afford to continue to offer health insurance by shifting costs to their employees. Would an increase in direct responsibility for costs cause patients to use health care more prudently? Or would these new benefit packages create financial barriers to needed care, especially for lower-income workers? The jury is still out on these questions, but the reality of slimmed-down, higher-deductible benefit packages is likely to be just around the corner in many of the major medical markets in the United States.

In this scenario the ethical goal of health plans must be to ensure that a core set of medically necessary services are unalterably included within their benefit packages. Health plans must also work with purchasers to create a selection of benefit packages that offers viable choices for the most financially vulnerable patients. One mechanism we saw of moderating the free play of market forces in benefit design is the use of a feedback loop between benefit design teams and the medical leadership of a health plan. The medical leadership can be given the organizational responsibility of making sure that benefit packages make sense and include necessary services and that they do not create untenable ethical dilemmas for coverage decisions should an individual need appropriate medical care but find the necessary services are not a covered benefit.

Technology Assessment

Technology assessment is often closely linked with coverage decisions in that the impetus for a formal technology assessment often comes first from a specific request for an individual patient to receive coverage for a new test or treatment. The central ethical obligations of technology assessment focus on the scientific rigor and transparency of the process used to evaluate the effectiveness of a medical service. Appropriate expertise is required in those appointed to examine the scientific literature. These individuals must also be free of any significant financial conflict of interest linked to their decisions. And the process they follow to render an assessment or a formal judgment of effectiveness must be clearly defined and followed consistently.

Coverage Decisions

The distinction between technology assessment and coverage decision making is subtle, yet quite important. In most health plans, technology assessment is performed by a small committee, sequestered from most other operational concerns. Technology assessment is "pure" and looks in a cool-headed fashion at the evidence; coverage decisions, on the other hand, are made in a messy, real world in which evidence must be considered in the context of competitors, legal risk, local physician skills, and the details of individual patient cases. The organization's own history of similar decisions in the past must be considered, along with the potential to create a new and possibly expensive precedent with every decision. Coverage decisions in small health plans may be made by a single medical director, but in larger health plans, the process often involves formal input from actuaries, sales and marketing managers, and benefit design staff. The raw material handed down by technology assessment is but a part of what feeds actual coverage decisions.

Our central ethical obligations for organizations in the area of coverage decisions emphasize transparency and disclosure. Certainly, coverage decisions should continue to be determined largely by the strength of the evidence of clinical effectiveness, tempered by the unique characteristics of each patient's situation. The internal process must be clinically informed, well organized, and free from significant conflict of interest. But the ethical dimensions of coverage decisions also include the critical phase of communication with patients and physicians about the rationale for a denial of coverage. This communication must be honest and forthright; it should convey the evidence and reasons that went into the ultimate decision. If costs or cost-effectiveness were a part of the decision, then this too should be acknowledged. And, in the face of a coverage denial, every attempt should be made to communicate with patient and physician regarding alternative means of caring for the patient. A denial-of-coverage decision cannot be allowed to be equated with abandonment. The obligations of the health plan to help facilitate the patient's care become greater following a denial of coverage, and this responsibility must be embraced by the organization. Concomitantly, the health plan should mark out the path toward benefit adjudication and make sure it is clear and unobstructed for the patient.

This collection of obligations may seem to set a very high standard for health care organizations. Attention to them all takes a lot of organizational focus and resources. But this is the ethical price of owning the determination of medical necessity.

Benefit Adjudication

Benefit adjudication shares with coverage decision making the ethical obligations necessary for any organizational process to be called consistent, fair, and transparent to outside observers. But because benefit adjudication is only used when patients have experienced the disappointment and disillusion of an initial denial of coverage, the steps necessary for building a trustworthy process represent an even greater challenge. The emphasis on transparency begins with an obligation of making the benefit adjudication process clear and unthreatening to patients and physicians. Decisions reached in benefit adjudication must also be made clear and their rationales made accessible to patients. But even if these elements of procedural justice are addressed, special attention must be paid to concerns about the trustworthiness of the individuals responsible for making benefit adjudication decisions. After all, health plan staff have already issued a denial of coverage. Who is it now who will serve on the "Supreme Court" that hears appeals? Systems should be in place to ensure that the review of coverage decisions is performed by individuals who are clinically informed and who can be indifferent to the financial ramifications of any decision for the health plan. This is the ethical obligation. Since it may well be impossible to create a robust internal benefit adjudication system in which decision makers have no vested interest in the outcome, patients should have ultimate recourse to a truly independent, external review body. As mentioned in the introduction to this chapter, external review has not proven to be a panacea for questions about the legitimacy of benefit adjudication. The ethical obligation of creating a system that is fair and will be perceived as trustworthy by patients, even if they are told "no," remains a challenge for all health-care organizations that interpret the boundaries between coverage and medical necessity.

EXEMPLARY PRACTICES

Within each piece of the medical policy-making machinery, there are inherent ethical tensions that must be resolved and core ethical obligations attendant upon their resolution. But it is often in the interaction of the different elements of medical policy that an organization's true ethical approach comes most to light. In many ways, the ethical legitimacy of medical policy depends on how the components function together in framing and reaching tough individual decisions. From our evaluation of the overall approach to medical policy at health plans and provider groups, we perceived three dominant approaches, each of which reflected deep cultural and historical features within the organizations. In presenting these approaches here, we purposely overemphasize the differences among them in order to frame the key paradigmatic choices available to health-care organizations in designing medical policy affecting the determination of medical necessity. In our formulation, these three approaches reflect differing views of the state of medical care, of physicians' skills and attitudes, and of patients' role in medical decisions. Building upon these different foundational attitudes, the three approaches can be seen to produce systems of medical policy determination that sit at different points on a spectrum from loose control over medical necessity and appropriateness to a form of tighter control. Within each of these different approaches resides the possibility of various exemplary practices in the determination of medical necessity.

The Doctor Is Right

In the first of these general approaches to medical policy, the organizations' culture, policies, and leadership all express an overriding belief that treating physicians are the sole arbiters of what a patient needs in a given circumstance. The underlying mantra is that health plans should, essentially, stay out of the way. According to this general view, physicians are universally beneficial agents who know the right thing to do for their patients; thus, the role of the health plan should be to get out of the way of the physician and the patient whenever possible. This view harkens back to the culture of indemnity insurance in which it was the insurer's role simply to verify that the service requested was a covered benefit and to leave all questions of the appropriate use of that service to the individual treating physician. Within this mindset, medical necessity and medical appropriateness therefore mean one and the same thing—the distinction is nearly meaningless.

Although there is no health plan whose characteristics match this accentuated picture, we did discover that some plans seem especially inspired by this general vision of the medical world and their role in it. Not surprisingly, we found that these health plans either had evolved from an historical base as a pure indemnity insurer or they had emerged from physician-led organizations with strong roots in the hospital community. Given their historical and cultural links to the model of physician-driven determinations of medical necessity, we examined what kinds of specific structures and processes these organizations had developed for medical necessity determination.

One example of a health plan that exemplifies this approach is the University of Pittsburgh Medical Center (UPMC) Health Plan. Its general philosophy is summed up in the first sentence of its enrollment decision guide for prospective members: "UPMC Health Plan is designed to set new standards for managed care—enabling caregivers to make the decision about members' health care." UPMC Health Plan was founded as an outgrowth of a provider organization centered in the hospitals and affiliates of the University of Pittsburgh. Initially, these hospitals and physician groups had come together in an effort to improve their efficiency and their bargaining position with external insurers. Later, they decided to create their own health plan as well. The health plan could help provide a more stable patient base for the hospitals and physicians and allow the provider group to compete directly with other insurers.

From its inception, therefore, UPMC Health Plan had been a junior partner within the overall UPMC Health System. It was the progeny of physician leaders seeking to support the clinical, academic, and economic interests of the leading medical institutions in the area. Given this history, UPMC Health Plan's culture is sharply defined: it exudes trust and confidence in its physicians and hospitals to practice cost-effective medicine. Physicians exercise their clinical freedom while remaining accountable for the rational use of practice profiles and other feedback to improve their clinical care. The health plan views its role as a source of information and data to help providers realize a hassle-free, yet cost-effective, vision of care.

Medical necessity is therefore conceptualized broadly at UPMC Health Plan; it is not seen as a tightly held commodity. At the time of our review, early in the growth and development phase of the plan, centralized medical policy was in a relatively early stage of development. Organizational focus and attention were on other priorities. Three years later, the plan would be fourth on the list of the 25 fastest growing health plans in the nation. With growth came an increase in preauthorization requirements, but relatively speaking, medical policy continued to have a somewhat limited profile within the organization, and the decisions about the appropriateness of specific tests and treatments in the care of individual patients remained largely at the discretion of individual providers.

When we visited UPMC Health Plan, the functions of technology assessment and benefit coverage decision making were not highlighted within the framework of the organization. The process for benefit adjudication had been closely regulated by the state, and, given the organizations' largely hands-off approach, it did not seem to be a prominent concern. Even UPMC Health Plan's clinical guidelines were used only as educational tools rather than as protocols for preauthorization or for determining post-hoc appropriateness for claims adjudication.

It is worth noting that the way that medical necessity determinations and medical policy in general were handled at UPMC Health Plan was not reflected in its formal definition of medical necessity. In 1999 UPMC Health Plan had been required to write an operational definition of medical necessity for state regulators in Pennsylvania. In this written definition, UPMC Health Plan reserved "the right to determine in its sole judgment whether a service is Medically Necessary and Appropriate." The plan's definition, of appropriate medical care includes language referring to benchmarks of scientific standards: [appropriate medical care is] provided in accordance with standards of good medical practice and consistent in type, frequency, and duration of treatment with scientifically based guidelines from medical research, or health care coverage organizations or governmental. . . ." According to these definitions, one might assume that UPMC Health Plan was similar to health plans that focused heavily on preauthorization and had a heavy-handed approach to medical necessity determination. But this is a good example of how the regulatory definitions of medical necessity can reveal very little about the true character of the medical policy apparatus and culture within a health plan. Medical necessity language usually preserves enough degrees of freedom for the development of any number of different approaches. At UPMC we found a clear and strong providercentric organizational culture, with its attendant loose system of organizational processes for medical necessity determination.

A good exmaple of how UPMC Health Plan sees its role at the interface between providers and medical necessity is its unusual special needs department. According to UPMC Health Plan's internal documents, this department had been created to "fulfill services that are not a covered benefit [but that] may have a positive impact on health care status." All of UPMC Health Plan's disease management nurses had been grouped together in this department to discuss special situations that might call for extraordinary organizational efforts. For example, at one time, breast pumps had not been a covered benefit, but when case managers saw the need for many mothers to use breast pumps in order to return to work, the case managers, as a team, obtained approval for benefit exceptions for all patients until the benefit design group could add breast pumps as a covered benefit.

Nurses working in the special needs department had also taken concerted action to help patients with asthma and other respiratory disorders during an unprecedented summer heat wave. Working with city officials, the nurses helped low-income health plan members obtain $200 city vouchers that could be used toward the purchase of air conditioners. These stories, and others, of pushing bureaucratic boundaries in order to pursue patients' needs beyond defined coverage boundaries were related with sincere pride. They spoke not only of the dedication of the individual nurses in this department but of one kind of exemplary organizational practice in managing the ethical tensions inherent in medical necessity determinations. UPMC Health Plan spent considerable organizational resources to ensure that its providers could get the services they wanted for their patients, even if those services weren't initially covered or weren't considered medically necessary.

Evidence Is King

In some health plans we visited, there emerged a different dominant theme: an almost canonical reverence for the potential of medical evidence to improve health care and to answer all difficult questions related to medical necessity. In this mindset, physicians—and patients—are perceived to be generally good and appropriate users of medical resources, and they lack only timely and accurate scientific information to achieve even better performance. Job 1 of the health plan is to apply evidence liberally, like a salve to a wound, to drive the health-care system toward this vision of better performance. Where there is excessive variation in health outcomes or utilization, where there is poor performance on preventive measures, where there are inappropriate gaps between knowledge and practice, the health plan should actively wield evidence-based measures to fix the problem. Good evidence will lead to better health outcomes and improved efficiency, which are viewed as nearly indivisible and mutually supportive. The belief is clear: better evidence, distributed more broadly among providers and patients and more effectively applied through population-based systems of care, will improve health and lower costs at the same time. If there is a problem, evidence is the answer.

This general philosophy often distinguishes itself by the fervor with which it believes that evidence-based information can guide physicians and patients toward medically appropriate care. A deep belief in the power of evidence, however, is only part of the picture. Allied to the belief in evidence is the faith that the best way to use evidence is to democratize it—to hand it over to providers and patients, who will then apply it with sovereignty in the office. This general view assumes that providers and patients will heed the evidence, apply it with appropriate sensitivity in the context of the individual patient's situation, and arrive at the best medical decisions without the need for supervision by the health plan. Recently, the Internet has caused an evolution in this philosophy toward including the patient ever more in the decision-making process, and an informed, engaged patient now finds a central position in an optimistic view that ideal care can be achieved through a participatory, evidence-based conversation between an individual patient and physician.

Although one can find echoes of this philosophy in most health plans, some plans seem to frame their entire approach to medical necessity and medical policy upon its foundation. The Group Health Cooperative of Puget Sound is one example of an archetypal health plan for which evidence is king.

Group Health has evolved significantly in the last decade from its roots as one of the earliest staff-model HMOs in the United States. New business ventures, contractual arrangements with providers, and organizational structures have arisen in the organization's attempt to compete in the marketplace. But within the culture of the organization, some things have apparently not changed that much from the early days of consumer power and social solidarity: "The vision is that the patient and physician will make the right decision and we won't need any oversight at all. The vision is one of shared decision making, with evidence playing a dominating, central role. We will provide tools to individualize care, not ration it. This is the core of our vision of population-based care." These comments by a senior Group Health medical director set forth the organization's basic vision of medical necessity determinations and medical policy.

Group Health has an almost evangelical belief in the role the organization plays in bringing evidence-based medical practice to as wide a population as possible. The well-known *Group Health Roadmaps*—rigorous, population-based clinical guidelines—are a testament to the way that Group Health incorporates a strong faith in evidence with respect for individual decision making. As it has for previous guideline efforts, Group Health committed significant organizational resources to the development and implementation of the new *Roadmaps*. These guidelines were explicitly meant to reshape the way that the entire health-care system was organized to care for patients with certain chronic conditions, such as diabetes mellitus and coronary artery disease. Part of the thrust of these guidelines was to increase the engagement of patients in their own care. The *Roadmap* initiatives were also intended to bring evidence-based guidelines to physicians in their offices and to support them in providing state-of-the-art clinical medicine to every Group Health patient.

In an organization where evidence has such influence, it is not surprising that Group Health has focused considerable thought and placed significant emphasis on the committees and processes responsible for benefit design, technology assessment, coverage decision making, and benefit adjudication. Group Health's conscious awareness of ethical issues surrounding these areas, as well as its organizational approach, can be seen quite clearly in its conceptualization of benefit design. At the time of our site visit, Group Health had approximately 850 different benefit plans, the variation being driven by the unique demands of individual employer-purchasers. In late 1999, as part of a general response to the increasing competitive forces calling for further benefit package variation, Group Health developed a statement of values and principles to guide health-care benefit plan design. This values statement was formally approved by the board of directors to guide the benefit design process. It is a striking document in its acknowledgement of ethical tensions inherent in benefit design and in its thoughtful approach to the delineation of values and principles to navigate these ethical tensions in the benefit design process.

The first value described in the document is that benefit designs should promote fair treatment of enrollees. This immediate, and abiding, focus on the enrollee helps set the tone for the entire values statement. The integrity of benefit packages in the face of competitive pressures to strip out certain benefits is an issue directly confronted within the document. Group Health states that it "recognizes the dilemma posed by high cost/low volume procedures and the potential impact on rates and competition. At the same time, there is recognition that one purpose of an organization like Group Health is to protect individuals from undue financial risk and provide a benefit package that is consistent with consumers' collective needs and desires."

The document goes on to outline other basic Group Health values and principles that should be incorporated in all benefit package designs. The document notes that there might be occasions of dynamic tension between the health plan's goals, principles and values, and marketing considerations. One of the more helpful aspects of this document is the way it not only delineates important values and principles but goes on to specify how they are directly applicable to the ethical tensions inherent in some plan design decisions. For instance, in discussing the Group Health principle of minimizing financial risk to enrollees, the document specifies that this principle bears directly on the design of co-payments in benefit plans. Group Health has a program of co-payment stop-loss provisions to protect individual patients from bearing extremely high costs due to the need for frequent physician visits. As the document makes clear, the goal behind this provision of ensuring low out-of-pocket costs for enrollees must be weighed against the potential for adverse selection in the insurance market.

Several other values and principles in the document are worth noting. Broadly stated here, as well, is the underlying faith in the role of evidence to guide the design of benefits: "Clinical evidence and scientific knowledge related to medical efficacy and appropriateness should guide benefit plan designs. Designs should allow Group Health to seek a leadership position in setting the standards of efficient and appropriate care and practice in the community." The document also notes that Group Health highly values prevention and screening: "Routine care, preventive care, and the promotion of health should be emphasized in the design of the health care benefit plan."

Linked closely to the process of benefit design is Group Health's approach to assessing new technologies and rendering coverage decisions based on a determination of medical necessity. Here again, Group Health is notable for the conscious attention given to ethical values and for its heavy reliance on medical evidence to clarify tough decisions. In the past, Group Health had a single committee responsible for two functions: (1) performing a technology assessment; and (2) making the ultimate decision on whether a new test or procedure would be covered. The health plan has now split these functions across two groups. First, to perform the technology assessment, the plan relies upon a medical technology assessment committee, or MTAC. The MTAC has broad representation from clinical and epidemiological experts and also includes a consumer member of the board of trustees.

The MTAC has an explicit three-phase process for technology assessment. First, there is a strict and rigorous evidence-based assessment of the effectiveness of a medical device or procedure. This evaluation applies the principles of evidence-based medicine while being conscious of the complications presented by limited evidence, strong advocacy by patients and providers, pressures to make decisions quickly, "the love of the marvelous," and the extra attention and pressure attendant with last-chance treatments for dying patients. The key elements of the MTAC process include: systematic strategies to obtain evidence; a formalized critical appraisal of that evidence; and a printed evidence summary that is handed off to the body responsible for making the ultimate coverage decision. The MTAC uses five formal evaluation criteria for judging the effectiveness of a medical technology. These five criteria were originally created by the Technology Evaluation Center (TEC), a program developed by the Blue Cross Blue Shield Association and administered in partnership with Kaiser Permanente:

- The technology must have the final approval from the appropriate government regulatory bodies, if applicable.

- The scientific evidence must permit conclusions concerning the effects of the technology on health outcomes.
- The technology must improve the net health outcome.
- The technology must be as beneficial as any established alternatives.
- The improvement must be attainable outside the investigational setting.

If the MTAC finds that the technology meets all five criteria, then the MTAC will judge the technology to be medically effective. As part of such a recommendation, the MTAC may include specific patient selection criteria.

Until recently, the MTAC was also responsible for the ultimate coverage decision for each technology that it judged to be effective. When it had the responsibility to make the ultimate coverage decision itself, the MTAC applied one final criterion: "The technology must represent an efficient use of limited resources." In deciding whether an effective technology represented an efficient use of resources, the MTAC considered the cost of the technology to the patient, the provider, and the health plan. Additionally, comparisons were made to the effectiveness and cost of currently provided and covered medical technologies in the same area. In the end, the MTAC would decide to cover only those technologies for which it made "both medical and economic sense" to pay. This level of honesty regarding the role of costs in coverage decisions is rare indeed within the competitive U.S. healthcare system.

As noted, Group Health eventually decided to separate the function of assessing effectiveness from the responsibility of making the ultimate coverage decision. Now the MTAC sends its assessment of effectiveness to a different group, called the Health Plan Medical Directors Group (HPMDG), that makes the coverage decision. This group is composed of senior medical directors and representatives from the key health plan departments. The HPMDG considers the evidence and assessment of MTAC as well as other factors such as community practices, cost, and patient or practitioner advocacy. As noted in its mission statement, the HPMDG ensures a balance between medical policy, medical efficacy, and market/environment realities. The HPMDG then reaches a decision to include or exclude the proposed new technology in the benefit.

The cumulative work of the MTAC and the HPMDG goes to support the development of a set of *clinical criteria* used by Group Health to make many day-to-day coverage decisions. These clinical criteria are used for preauthorization purposes to determine medical necessity and can serve as the basis for Group Health issuing a notice of noncoverage for a procedure or service. Group Health makes all of its clinical criteria available on the Internet for its physicians, who are actively encouraged to visit the website. As in other areas, Group Health expresses through its words and its actions a profound confidence in the ability of evidence, openly discussed and rigorously evaluated, to serve as a common guide to medically appropriate, highly cost-effective care.

The Health Plan at the Center

In the third major approach to medical necessity determination, evidence remains closely scrutinized and highly valued, but the role of the health plan in bringing the benefits of evidence to its members is conceptualized somewhat differently. An important way to understand the distinction is to consider the health plan–physician-patient relationship. In health plans such as Group Health, where the dominant organizational culture, and many of its structures, still resonate with its history as a staff-model HMO, there is a natural congruence between the health plan, its physicians, and its members. Within this kind of health plan, many of the physicians see only Group Health members, and the historical roots of the staff-model HMO have retained an especially loyal core of members with whom the health plan has a special relationship.

Far different is the situation of health plans built upon large, diffuse networks of affiliated, but strikingly independent, physician practices. With a structure that reflects the effort to offer more choice to members, these health plans lack a history of a more cohesive organizational structure directly linking the insurance function with the direct provision of health care. Physicians affiliated with these health plans most often have practices that see patients with many different insurance plans, and most physicians are unlikely to feel a special relationship with only one of the health plans with which they contract. In some parts of the country, such as California, physicians have joined together for the purposes of contracting, thereby creating another level of administration. These physicians' groups, or independent practice associations, were created to help put medical decision making back in the hands of practicing physicians. Physicians may have relationships with multiple physicians' groups and, as a result, multiple insurance companies and health maintenance organizations. For health plans, these multiple relationships can result in a sense of physician indifference. Clinical guidelines, formularies, disease management efforts, and other attempts to reach out and mold clinical practice through the use of evidence may be discounted by physicians as only contributing to the avalanche of paper they receive from insurers. Information overload may lead physicians to ignore health plan attempts to improve the quality and efficiency of care. And the diffuse network of independent practices increases the chances that local variations in practice styles will flourish. Meanwhile, enrollees who select this kind of health plan mirror the physicians and are less likely to view themselves as part of a unique cooperative or community.

Health plans with this history, structure, and membership face greater challenges than staff- and group-model HMOs in implementing evidence-based tools effectively throughout their physician networks. While working hard to get evidence-based tools to all their physicians, one common organizational strategy has been to complement this effort with a more centralized role for the health plan itself in determining medical appropriateness. Information and requests from participating physicians flow to the health plan at the center, where the health plan serves as an important anchor and often applies evidence-based tools itself in the effort to improve the quality and efficiency of care received by its members. In years past, health plans along this model often served as the archetypal obstructive, bureaucratic HMO, with the full complement of infamous 1–800 numbers, burdensome administrative hoops, and bean counters making clinical decisions. Other network-model health plans that contracted primarily through capitation agreements with large physicians' groups chose to delegate to these groups many elements of medical policy and utilization review. But even in these situations, the health plans exert guidance over medical necessity determination through their own medical policies. Today health plans offering broad physician networks with increased choice of physicians and less vertical integration of care have come to dominate the U.S. health-care system. Even venerable staff-model HMOs have merged or changed to include broader and looser physician networks. Nearly every health plan now needs to know how best to frame its approach to medical necessity and how to create and implement medical policy when the health plan is at the center of a wide, diffuse, and loosely integrated system.

At Health Net of California, medical policy is big—big conceptually, big organizationally, and big literally, as is evident when lifting its three-pound, 1184-page *Guide to Evidence-Based Medicine*, a compendium of utilization management criteria, clinical practice guidelines, and technology assessment that was sent to all providers in late 2000 (Health Net, 2000). This compendium was the latest in a growing effort by Health Net to share with its providers what had once been viewed internally as a proprietary asset. In the past, medical policies not available to providers or the public were used as part of preauthorization and utilization review to define criteria for coverage. Today, Health Net has turned that notion on its head and is seeking to open up to providers the content of medical policies that do everything from suggesting general prevention guidelines to delineating the exact criteria for coverage for specific tests, procedures, and treatments. The black box is no more. Health Net's goal is to make medical policy excellently, to share it freely, to use it to improve the cost-effectiveness of care, and, ultimately, to win over practicing physicians and patients by the power of evidence marshaled into magisterial form by the health plan.

Health Net's *Guide* thus represents a forceful, state-of-the-art attempt to define the clinical boundaries of covered care. Within this vision, there is no distinction between medical necessity and medical appropriateness. Medical policy is both broad enough and detailed enough to subsume both. In the words of Health Net's own description, medical policy "identifies experimental status, written research protocols, appropriate clinical application, efficacy, safety, research findings, and medical consensus regarding medical technology" (Health Net, 2000, pp. 300–1). Since medical policy is so encompassing, Health Net is very attentive to defining the boundary between issues of medical necessity and issues of benefit coverage.

In fact, a striking feature of the *Guide* is the clarity and consistency with which it defines terms, assigns responsibilities, and seeks to separate the issues of benefit coverage decisions and medical necessity. Benefit coverage decisions at Health Net were described to us as having nothing to do with determining medical necessity, but are instead matters of interpreting the limits of specific contract language in the benefit package. Health Net medical leaders see this distinction as central to their vision of medical policy. Medical necessity is a matter isolated from other organizational concerns, solely determined by evidence of clinical effectiveness. It is as black and white as the medical policy printed in the *Guide*. Neither costs nor cost-effectiveness are to be considered, for in Health Net's way of thinking, this would contaminate what should be a purely scientific judgment. As is evident, we found at Health Net no corollary at all to Group Health's approach of determining that a medical service was medically necessary only if it made "medical and economic sense."

The broad effort represented by Health Net's *Guide* to share medical policy with providers should not conceal the central role that Health Net retains in developing and applying evidence-based medical policies. The culture within Health Net is not that of a passive partner. Health Net believes that it adds tremendous value by staying at the center, being the creator of policy and also the conduit through which practice decisions for individual patients must flow to receive coverage. As described in the *Guide*, "Attending providers are exclusively responsible for making all medical determinations and treatment decisions. However, payment for rendered services will be conditioned on Health Net's subsequent review and determination of consistency with professionally recognized standards of practice, benefit structure, and Health Net's medical policies." Words such as these convey the reality that Health Net has most assuredly not given up its control over medical necessity determinations. But Health Net believes it can retain control while simultaneously sharing the information that could be used to "game" the system. Health Net is trusting its providers with the keys to the previously locked box of coverage determination.

The introduction to the *Guide* lays out in detail the different elements of how the organization frames and develops medical policy. Given Health Net's attention to the procedure of creating medical policy, it is worth reviewing its description. The *Guide* has three components:

1. Clinical practice guidelines directed toward the Primary Care Physician (PCP) that outlines best practice for specific disease or disorder processes. Practice guidelines are derived primarily from specialty medical consensus statements and position papers.
2. Criteria sets that outline medically necessary indications for specific procedures, services, drugs, and supplies.

3. Technology assessments that include research information, Federal Drug Administration approvals, national standards, etc. Technology assessments include only those technologies, drugs, or procedures that are currently considered to be experimental/investigational in nature.

Medical policies originate and evolve under the direction of the Health Net medical policy department. The department consists of a full-time dedicated staff of three registered nurses (medical policy managers). In the development of medical policy documents, the medical policy department:

- Performs the literature search, including sources such as National Library of Medicine, government agencies (e.g., FDA, National Institutes of Health, Center of Disease Control and Prevention), and nationally recognized medical-specialty associations.
- Reviews the procedure or service to determine if it is considered investigational/experimental.
- Seeks input from internal departments (e.g., pharmacy, medical management, legal) and Health Net committees (e.g., legislative).
- Requests physician input from Health Net medical directors, participating physician groups and direct network physicians, and Health Net physician specialty committees.
- Develops a draft policy.

Following this process, the medical policy manager drafts or revises the policy based on the research and comments from all reviewers. The draft policy is submitted to Health Net's Evidence-Based Medicine Committee for review and formal approval. Membership of this committee includes 12 physicians from participating medical groups, representing each region of the health plan, and 3 Health Net medical directors. Approved medical policies are distributed to all providers through the policy manual, which, in addition to hard copy, is distributed via CD-ROM format and is now available on the Internet for all Health Net providers. All utilization management criteria sets and technology assessments are formally reviewed and updated annually, while clinical practice guidelines are reviewed on an every-two-year basis.

The approach to medical policy exemplified at Health Net uses evidence in an even more detailed fashion than does that at Group Health. By exhaustively defining the medical necessity of many tests and treatments, Health Net creates a tighter vision of appropriate care and criteria for coverage. At the center of a widespread and diverse network of providers, this is one way to manage care, to bring the added value of evidence-based medicine to all the health plan's members. Medical policy exercised in this fashion is the dominant approach used by national, for-profit health plans. When medical policy is developed by broad groups of clinicians and other stakeholders, when it is implemented with full disclosure to physicians, and when it is partnered with robust mechanisms for benefit adjudication, this approach offers another potential model for exemplary organizational practice.

LESSONS LEARNED

Without exception, the medical leaders within each organization in the BEST project recognized medical necessity determinations as ethically challenging. The conflicts between patients' hopes, physicians' autonomy, often murky evidence, and pressures to control costs were not going to go away. There were no naïve assertions that conflict-free processes could ever be developed, only a frank realization that no matter how hard they tried, they would be left making many difficult decisions in particular cases. The tumultuous wrestling match with organized medicine over the power to determine medical necessity was also viewed as likely to continue. Yet, cautious optimism was also universal. It was clear to these organizations that a new era had already begun. Secret, proprietary processes and criteria for making medical necessity determinations had undermined trust in managed care, and the public backlash had helped to blow open the doors on this once tightly held corporate practice. As with other forms of information in the emerging Internet age, medical necessity criteria could no longer be held captive. In place of the old approach, there was emerging a new consensus that evidence-based tools could be freely shared with physicians and patients. If medical necessity were not to be handed back to physicians and patients, at least it could be discussed openly without leading to the financial ruin of the organization.

And so, perhaps the most dominant common feature of the exemplary medical necessity practices we found was a commitment, permeating these organizations, to improve the openness of decision-making processes and results. The Internet was viewed as an extraordinary medium for sharing information universally and inexpensively. The only questions seemed to be how fast the organizations could get the information on the Web.

The practices we singled out as exemplary also reflected a deep belief in the use of evidence to improve the quality and efficiency of care. All the organizations in the BEST project touted their use of evidence, but each created its own unique method for gathering evidence, weighing it in relation to the values of various stakeholders, and setting that evidence within medical policy and other organizational methods to control the delivery and coverage of care. Given these variations, it seemed clear that what we considered to be exemplary practices to determine medical necessity could arrive at different conclusions regarding coverage for any particular service or technology. We consider it vitally important that exemplary medical necessity processes include formal mechanisms for trying to benchmark decisions internally for consistency and externally for validity against those of other health plans. But the absence of perfect uniformity means that, inevitably, a patient in one health plan might be allowed coverage for a new treatment when an identical patient, a member of a different health plan, would be denied coverage for that same treatment. Although such differing health plan decisions fly in the face of the desire for a justice that would treat like patients the same, we believe that the inexactitude of scientific information, combined with local variations in experience and quality of providers, will mean that ethically legitimate decision-making processes will sometimes arrive at different outcomes.

Another feature common to the exemplary practices we observed was the degree of integration across the different elements of medical policy. Each organization had a carefully thought-out plan, usually formalized through interlocking committee memberships, to link benefit design, technology assessment, coverage decision making, and benefit adjudication. Each organization had stories to tell of how important it was that this integration functioned well. When it did not, serious inconsistencies could arise that led to holes in benefit packages, patient and physician confusion, coverage decisions lacking in reliability, and systematic errors in billing and benefit adjudication. A passion for consistency, rooted in the use of evidence and the documentation of decision rationales, motivated all of the organizations that had outstanding integration across medical policy functions. In the best systems we also found constant evidence of attention to the external as well as the internal "customer." For example, exemplary practices all included mechanisms for rapid back-and-forth communication between medical leadership and members of the health plan's benefit design group in order to avoid the creation of medically unsound benefit packages. The importance of attending to external customers was also made clear by internal benefit adjudication systems that paid primary attention to meeting the needs of patients and physicians. To achieve this end, exemplary practices often included outreach efforts to help guide patients through the maze of adjudication procedures.

As notable as are the common themes and features of exemplary practices, so too are important differences among the three major approaches we identified. For instance, medical necessity determination, along the general outlines of the approach we call "The Doctor is Right," lowers the profile of the health plan and may appeal to many physicians and patients who want as much freedom as possible to determine what care is indicated for the individual patient. Such an approach may lesson administrative costs related to the development of clinical guidelines and the application of preauthorization and utilization review criteria. But in many health-care markets the risk is that physicians will not manage care in a cost-effective manner, especially if they do not share any financial risk with the health plan. Variation in the quality of care may also be substantial.

If we take the second approach, in which "Evidence is King," success is likely to depend on how effective the evidence actually is in molding the behavior of physicians. Of course, in the ideal world, all physicians and patients would receive and use individualized evidence together for superior, tailored, evidence-based medicine. Where the evidence is applied through an organizational structure and with the supports to turn knowledge into action, this approach will succeed. On the other hand, most health plans cannot seek to realize this vision through a tightly integrated delivery system. And many health plans do not have the resources to try to implement evidence-based practice through a more diffuse delivery network. As many academic experiments have shown, it is not hard for evidence by itself to fail to change physician and patient behavior.

There is another caveat about the widely held faith in the power of evidence to solve medical necessity problems. Evidence is imperfect; it rarely comes in black-and-white clarity. The deeper problems faced by the health plans in our study have been in weighing of evidence amid the varying perspectives and values of different stakeholders. Is Viagra a treatment for a serious condition that affects the quality of life as much as congestive heart failure, or is it an optional tonic to boost one's lifestyle? Data on clinical outcomes, risks, and costs alone will not answer this question nor lead to an obvious answer regarding coverage for Viagra. Exemplary practices of medical necessity determination, no matter how well grounded in evidence, must also contain mature methods for seeking out stakeholder values and integrating them in the decision-making process.

For the third general approach, "Health Plan at the Center," health plans would seem to have the advantage of a centralized process that could apply the rigor of evidence across a diffuse network to maintain high levels of quality and cost-effectiveness. The more comprehensive and detailed the medical policy is, the more uniform the process of medical necessity determination would become. And through the Internet, the details of medical policy could be made available to all parties, perhaps increasing the buy-in of physicians and patients and, at the very least, enhancing the legitimacy of requiring physicians and their patients to understand and play by the rules. When done right, medical appropriateness and necessity would merge into a single, concrete entity. This approach, however, requires exquisite sensitivity to the transparence of the processes through which medical policies are created. Is the evidence gathered in an unbiased fashion? Are the right physicians included in the process? Are patients included? In the exemplary practices we identified, there was great sensitivity to these questions, but it was still too early to know whether physicians and the public would share in the health plans' faith in the ethical legitimacy of their decision-making processes. The health plan at the center still runs a greater risk of being perceived as a blocker of treatment rather than a facilitator of improved care. Not unaware of this risk, exemplary practices in this model placed special emphasis on communication with physicians on benefit questions, and they developed sophisticated methods to ensure that patients had rapid access to external review for any adverse medical necessity decision.

Each health plan, with its own unique history, structure, and culture, will find many options for constructing an exemplary practice to determine medical necessity. Despite intense regulatory interest, there are likely to remain great opportunities for organizations to exceed minimum requirements and to build practices of true ethical excellence. The future will only place greater emphasis on the ethical features of medical necessity, coverage decisions, and medical policy. As technology continues to provide new, effective treatments, and as the U.S. population ages, decisions about what is medically necessary are likely to become even more pervasive and difficult. The same trends and problems will afflict the national health care systems of other countries. It is our belief that exemplary practices to determine medical necessity will mark the most successful health plans and health care systems of the future. Tough decisions will need to be made. Tough decisions made with high ethical standards will command public approval and commercial success. From the experience and insights of the organizations in the BEST project, we hope that other organizations, regulators, and policy advocates will discern elements of exemplary practices in medical necessity determination that will guide the positive evolution of all health-care organizations responsible for caring for patients within a budget.

NOTE

1. This synopsis draws on material presented in Bergthold (1995) and Rosenbaum and colleagues (1999), but relies particularly on the excellent review of the history of the concept of medical necessity contained in a journal article by Eddy (1996).

6

THE CARE OF
VULNERABLE POPULATIONS

Deborah Jones is a single mother of three children: 5, 3, and 1 years
old. She burst into tears in the pediatrician's office when the doctor reminded her that the two younger children were behind in their
immunizations. Ms. Jones had been worried about this, but she
already had missed too much work caring for the kids when they
were ill, and she was afraid she would lose her job (and thus her
health insurance) if she took any additional time for their well-child
care appointments. Unfortunately, there didn't seem to be an easy
solution to her problems. She left the office with a fistful of new
weekday appointments with the pediatrician, but she had already
decided that she would have to try another option: she would take
the kids to the emergency room on the weekend with "sore throats"
and hope they could get their vaccinations then.

Yefimia Shlapakova is a 63-year-old woman who recently immi-
grated to the United States from Russia. She arrived with empty
bottles of "heart" pills labeled in Russian. Having qualified for a
state managed care Medicaid program, she was taken to her first
doctor's appointment by her nephew, who had been in the United
States for three years but still did not speak English well. Ner-
vous yet proud, Ms. Shlapakova spoke forcefully in her native
language to her doctor, Dr. Crocker, who smiled and turned to
the nephew for a full translation but got only a fraction of what
the patient said. The physical examination soon revealed, however, that Ms. Shlapakova had severe hypertension and showed signs
suggesting chronic renal failure as well. Ms. Shlapakova nodded
affirmatively, and pointed meaningfully to her empty pill bottles.
Her nephew said these medicines were the only ones that had ever
worked for her and that other hypertension medicines made her very
sick. Ms. Shlapakova made clear by her gestures that she would
only take the medicines she was familiar with. Dr. Crocker picked
up the empty bottles, squinted at them, and sighed. Even when he
had Ms. Shlapakova read the names out loud, he didn't recognize
any of them. Dr. Crocker stepped out of the exam room, called
the Russian interpreter's office located in the clinic, and asked
that an interpreter be sent over to help sort things out. Dr. Crocker
knew that the Russian interpreters always took new patients like
Ms. Shlapakova under their wing, established one-on-one longitudinal relationships with them, and quickly became an integral part

of their health-care team. This program had worked so well that Dr. Crocker had come to love getting new Russian patients. He had even learned how to say hello, goodbye, and thank you in Russian, much to the delight of his patients.

One of the ethical challenges health plans in the United States must confront is how to adhere to the traditional medical value of caring for the sickest and most vulnerable patients while shepherding limited resources for an entire population. This challenge is made all the more difficult by the fact that health plans must compete for economic survival in a system that offers greater profits to organizations that spend less on care. And vulnerable patients cost more. From the vignettes at the beginning of this chapter, for instance, it is clear that Deborah Jones and her children are not only more challenging to care for than most families but also are at greater risk of seeking expensive care. Yefimia Shlapakova will love the interpreter-advocate program established by her health plan, but the program is likely to be quite costly and may not pay for itself by reducing unnecessary clinic and hospital visits. In some ways, therefore, health-care organizations in the United States cannot escape at least an unconscious ambivalence about welcoming patients from vulnerable populations and spending money to improve their care. This tension is readily apparent in the distinction between the quiet pride that many organizations take in their special disease-management programs for complex patients, and the very public television commercials for the same health plans that feature young, active, and healthy adults wooing similar people to join up. The goal of taking excellent care of vulnerable populations duels daily with the perceived risks of *adverse selection*. Health plans embrace the idea of caring for vulnerable patients; they just want to make sure that they don't wind up with too many of them.

Who are the vulnerable patients in the U.S. health-care system? Certainly, individuals without health insurance are vulnerable, and any serious illness brings its own existential vulnerability to every patient. Nevertheless, physicians and health-care organizations have traditionally thought of certain groups as facing special and inherent barriers to receiving appropriate health care. Groups that are frequently considered vulnerable in this regard include the disabled, poor, non-English-speaking, mentally ill, elderly, or very young. These groups may not have equal access to care and are also more likely to experience poor coordination of care, medical error, and other unintended consequences of a fragmented health care system. Since the health care system is now dominated by large organizations, there is also a new way to capture the concept of vulnerability: individuals are vulnerable if they have any reason to be poor navigators of complex organizational processes.

Federal and state legislation prohibits health plans from systematically excluding patients on the basis of race, socioeconomic background, or health behaviors. Health plans are free, however, to decide the extent to which they will participate in public programs such as Medicaid and Medicare, which serve the poor, elderly, and disabled. Private health plans in the United States have had a stormy relationship with Medicaid and Medicare. The patients in these programs are often chronically ill and may have a combination of factors that make them among the most complex and challenging patients to take care of. In other words, they are vulnerable and can be very expensive. For many health plans, the ethical tension of caring for vulnerable populations came to a head during the late 1990s when growing operational deficits resulted in difficult and very public decisions to pull back and offer insurance only to Medicaid and Medicare patients who lived in specific geographic areas where reimbursement from state and federal governments fully covered expenses. Many health plans were forced to reexamine the viability of their organizational commitment to caring for those most in need.

Beyond questions regarding the scope of including vulnerable populations within a health plan lie additional ethical issues of how much to invest in special programs for their care. Ethical excellence lies in the combination of a sophisticated commitment to the care of vulnerable populations and the organizational creativity and innovation applied to the special problems faced by these patients. In this chapter we will examine the outlines of several exemplary approaches that have made this combination work well in competitive markets.

ETHICAL VALUES AND CENTRAL ETHICAL OBLIGATIONS

Health care organizations face difficult, pressing value conflicts in many aspects of caring for vulnerable populations. The moral obligation to take special care of vulnerable members of the population grows out of the value of communal solidarity—caring for a community as a whole, including all of its members. Just as the virtuous individual physician should treat all patients who need care, with special compassion and advocacy for the most vulnerable, so by extension, should health-care organizations share this value. Certain U.S. health-care organizations are more likely than others to feel a true obligation of communal solidarity. As opposed to national health plans, health plans founded on a specific geographic basis and those that emerge out of physician–hospital organizations are more likely to explicitly identify with the defined population of a community, including all of its most vulnerable members. In addition, not-for-profit health-care organizations have a more explicit obligation to serve the interests of their local communities and may translate this obligation into a deeper commitment to care for vulnerable populations. Other health-care organizations may have an explicit religious or other basis for their commitment to serving the neediest members of the community.

Solidarity as a value presumes a compassionate emotional bond between all members of a community. In its European conception, solidarity includes ideals of group obligation, mutuality, and social feeling. Some have argued that solidarity is foreign to American culture, that Americans tend to reduce solidarity to dispassionate claims of justice (Baker, 2001). The American philosopher John Rawls, for example, developed out of considerations of justice his famous *difference principle*, a principle of justice that prioritizes allocation in favor of the least well off (Rawls, 1971).

Whether the ethical value supporting care of vulnerable populations is based on the emotional conceptions of solidarity or on refined philosophical principles of justice, the moral obligation of health-care organizations is clear. But that is not to say that there are no competing ethical values that bring into question what the level and method of commitment to vulnerable populations should be. One competing value is found in the ideal of stewardship: the value of using shared medical resources wisely to maximize the health of the population. The allocation of significant resources to the most vulnerable patients may not, from a utilitarian perspective, lead to the aggregate maximization of health. Perhaps other, less vulnerable, patients would benefit more from a defined amount of medical care than would the neediest patients. This tension between the option of allocating resources to help those most disadvantaged and the option of allocating resources to maximize average health outcomes is one of the recognized unsolved rationing problems (Daniels and Sabin, 2002). And, as we have shown in previous chapters, this inherent ethical tension is thrown into even sharper contrast when the organization seeking to balance these values must do so while competing against other health care organizations in the market. The value of organizational success in the market is often demeaned as greediness or overconcern with profitability. While, in some instances, this accusation may be valid, in reality, an unarticulated but legitimate goal of almost all organizations is to remain in existence. Indeed, any health care organization must remain solvent to continue its mission of providing health care. As we were told, "No margin, no mission."

These competing ethical values form the basis for considering a health-care organization's approach to caring for vulnerable populations. As in the other ethical domains, our list of central ethical obligations emphasizes procedural elements of policy and decision making, supported by several broad normative obligations (see Table 6–1).

EXEMPLARY PRACTICES

Through our field studies we identified three primary conceptions of how organizations framed their commitment to vulnerable populations. These general conceptions helped organizations build a consistent internal approach to difficult decisions in which care of vulnerable populations had to be balanced against stewardship and financial profitability.

Table 6–1. Central ethical obligations for the care of vulnerable populations

1. Include an explicit commitment to the care of vulnerable populations in statements of organizational goals.
2. Demonstrate a broad understanding of health in social terms.
3. Have an overarching goal of sustaining the dignity of individuals under the care and protection of the organization.
4. Use specific financial strategies, such as cross-subsidization across business lines, to support the care of vulnerable populations.
5. Create organizational decision-making processes that encourage input and broad deliberation from multiple stakeholders whenever the organization must address the tension between values of caring for vulnerable populations, stewardship of resources, and organizational profitability.
6. Create delivery system structures and programs that consciously address the special needs of vulnerable populations.
7. Have specific mechanisms for outreach to get the input of vulnerable populations on the design of programs serving their needs.

In the first, the care of vulnerable populations was viewed as nothing more than one line of business for the organization. Although some special consideration might be given to the idea of serving the neediest patients, the overriding message was "Each tub on its own bottom." (This was another competitive-market pearl of wisdom we learned during our investigation. It means that each line of business has to make business sense for the organization; each has to be independently profitable.) Should the organization serve patients in Medicare or Medicaid programs? According to this concept, the answer must be one of dollars and cents. Short term losses that have the potential to grow into long-term losses must be avoided if the organization is to compete effectively in the market. This is not to say the organization would shirk its fair share of vulnerable patients. But unless the care of these patients brought profit to the organization, the right thing to do was to stay away.

A second conception of an organizational approach to the care of vulnerable populations is that of commitment to a specific, geographically defined community. Some health plans have roots that link them indelibly with a state or defined region. For such organizations, the idea of an unswerving commitment to vulnerable populations within their geographical domain is natural and compelling. Interesting strains can be seen within geographically defined health plans that begin to expand beyond their core membership areas. The commitment to the care of vulnerable populations in newer markets is unlikely to ever feel quite the same, but the idea of having two different ethical standards for similar patients leaves decision makers noticeably uncomfortable. Over time, the organization will either pull back into its original geographic area or slowly evolve its culture to find a new understanding of its commitment to vulnerable populations wherever they may be.

The third conception of how to ground an approach to the care of vulnerable populations is exemplified by religious health-care organizations. As we have seen in the case of Holy Cross Health System, organizations may locate their entire mission within the value of caring for the most vulnerable. For such organizations, business considerations and profitability are still quite important, but there is less a sense of balancing ethical values and more of crafting a business strategy that fully supports the priority given by the organization to the care of vulnerable patients.

Even among health-care organizations with similar general conceptions of their commitment to vulnerable populations, there can be a great deal of variation in how organizations define and operationalize their actual programs of care. These variations hold important ethical ramifications themselves and are worthy of close examination. In our field studies, we found that one key operational decision seemed to determine much of the character and structure of an organization's care programs: whether to "carve in" or "carve out." *Carving in* meant that the organization would rely on its own internal resources to provide care to vulnerable members. *Carving out*, on the other hand, meant it had chosen to contract with outside organizations with special expertise in working with particular vulnerable populations.

We also found that certain common themes were apparent in the operational approaches taken by organizations expressing a commitment to care of vulnerable populations. One such theme is "making the most of what is required." In many cases, organizations are required by state law to provide a particular type of service for vulnerable patients. These organizations developed exemplary practices by seeking to achieve the spirit of the law, rather than trying to meet the legal requirement in some minimal way. Another important theme is the willingness to engage in an iterative process to arrive at good solutions for practical problems; many of the most successful practices we examined evolved through trial and error.

And finally, we found that organizations with success in caring for vulnerable members of the population had learned to "to meet the population where they are." These organizations engaged vulnerable populations through aggressive outreach efforts, and, metaphorically, met them where they were by appreciating their unique cultural and structural barriers to accessing care. In the specific organizational examples discussed below, we describe how various exemplary programs for the care of vulnerable populations express and realize these themes.

"Carving In" the Care of Vulnerable Populations

BlueCross BlueShield of Tennessee (BCBST), a not-for-profit insurer in Tennessee, has an extremely interesting and well-thought-out approach to caring for members of vulnerable populations. BCBST's history in this area and its current policies illustrate success in achieving a number of the central ethical obligations in this domain: a broad understanding of health in social terms, an organizational structure that acknowledges the special needs of vulnerable populations, and specific outreach mechanisms to elicit input from members of vulnerable populations.

Despite having no previous experience with vulnerable populations, BCBST chose a "carve-in" model when it began insuring vulnerable members of the population with the establishment of TennCare in January 1994. The TennCare population consists of all Medicaid-eligible patients and those who are not eligible but are deemed uninsurable by certain specific criteria. This is a difficult population to manage. One problem is communication since there is a 30% illiteracy rate in the state of Tennessee. The population is split between rural and urban settings where different strategies for population management are needed.

Because of its large provider network, BCBST was pressured by the state to participate in TennCare when the program was being launched. The program was hotly debated, and the legislation establishing TennCare was finally passed a mere three months before the program was scheduled to begin. Thus, BCBST had only three months' notice before taking on approximately 200,000 new members, all of whom needed to be assigned to primary care managers (PCMs). Because there was no time to build a separate provider network for TennCare, BCBST did what the state had counted on them to do: they unilaterally altered their provider contracts so that every BCBST provider automatically became a provider for TennCare. Not surprisingly, the provider community vehemently opposed this action; providers had not been offered any voice in this decision or in the TennCare fee schedule. The administrative conscription of providers into the TennCare network, known locally as the "cram-down," had a large, negative impact on BCBST's relationships with the provider community. Many providers resigned entirely from BCBST's panel; the network shrunk from approximately 9,000 to a low of approximately 3,000. BCBST worked very hard during 1994 to build its provider network back up to approximately 6,000.

When BCBST began its TennCare business, the insurer was quite concerned about TennCare's potential to drain the ongoing profitable parts of the business. Consequently, the TennCare operations were established as an entirely separate unit within the health plan. BCBST's agreement with the state was that it would begin its participation in TennCare in the preferred provider organization (PPO) model that existed and that, by January 1997, it would change to operate as an HMO. This commitment was made despite the fact that BCBST had no experience with the HMO model and limited experience caring for vulnerable populations.

By the summer of 1995, the TennCare program was perceived to be a terrible problem for BCBST. It was projected to lose $40 million that year, and little progress had been made towards establishing an HMO framework for care. BCBST began hiring some outside leaders for the TennCare unit with experience and expertise in HMOs; these individuals joined some talented individuals from within the organization to build BlueCare, the TennCare HMO. The development team was given access to significant financial resources. The team built a close working relationship of interdependence in which all members were educated about all the functions and responsibilities of each team member. Those who were involved in this effort likened it to working in a small, entrepreneurial start-up organization.

The task was to build an HMO program to serve the TennCare population. The team realized that they needed to create a data-driven, evidence-based system. They needed all aspects of the operation to be closely integrated: medical management, claims, customer service, and compliance. In mid-1995, there was no information systems infrastructure to support this close integration; there was only a database to pay claims. One of the early, vital tasks was to create an information systems infrastructure to support the entire operation. Another important task was to re-shape the relationship with the provider network. The most basic aspect of that change was to begin credentialing providers, a practice, previously unheard of in Tennessee, that generated significant resistance.

The experience of the team that built BlueCare was unique within BCBST. Being a separate entity freed it from much of the bureaucracy of the large organization. It also afforded team members the opportunity for experimentation with new management strategies. Since the Tennessee health-care market had been, and remains to this day, relatively free from managed care, the TennCare HMO has served as an experimental model for the introduction of managed care into BCBST and into Tennessee. Within BCBST, BlueCare is viewed as a laboratory in which ideas are piloted. One of the most successful strategies BlueCare has devised is to divide the state into regions and to organize all aspects of operations by region so there is an integrated team for each part of the state. BCBST is now in the process of expanding the most successful aspects of BlueCare into the other lines of business in the organization.

Since the beginning of the program, the philosophy of the BlueCare staff has been that the care provided for TennCare members should be the same quality as that received by any BCBST member. This goal must be achieved, however, within a fixed budget not determined by BCBST. The BlueCare staff uses disease management programs to provide quality care in a cost-efficient manner. Because of a limited budget, only specific, highly targeted interventions are used. The interventions are usually pilot-tested in one or two regions, and their degree of success is evaluated within a relatively short time.

One of the difficulties in working with the TennCare population is maintaining an accurate database and finding ways to be in contact with members of the plan. The BlueCare staff has found that a large percentage of their members have phones, either residential or cellular. BlueCare has begun making so-called outbound calls to new members who enroll; they take the opportunity to orient the member to his or her benefits, explain how BlueCare works, and have the member select a primary care provider. BlueCare then provides the primary care provider with a list of patients, their current addresses and phone numbers, and information as to which children need immunizations that month. BlueCare also contacts *presumptive eligibles*, women who have had positive pregnancy tests at the county health department, and they connect these women to providers of prenatal care quickly. (If BlueCare were to wait for the state bureaucracy to identify these women and enroll them, there would be a long lag time before they began receiving prenatal care.)

BlueCare has invested an enormous amount of time and energy in trying to serve its members effectively. These efforts have been focused on advocacy and outreach. The philosophy of this program was to ally with community contacts that already had the trust of the people covered by TennCare. The outreach team contacted social service agencies, family resource centers, county health departments, and tenants' associations. They learned quickly that subtle characteristics of their approach, even how health plan representatives were dressed, influenced the reception they received in the community. They began by bringing small gifts, such as pens and mugs bearing the BlueCare logo. They did not initially ask the community contacts for assistance; rather, they offered their assistance with any problems people were experiencing with BlueCare. They also provided assistance with community problems unrelated to health care. Gradually, they built relationships with opinion leaders in the communities and a reputation as individuals who cared and an organization that could be trusted.

BlueCare staff members actively continue to maintain these relationships. They also rely on their community contacts to support BlueCare and BlueCare-related events. One focus of efforts is to ensure that all new members attend an orientation. Attendance is facilitated by holding the events in housing developments where people live, using door prizes and giveaways such as $50 off a month's rent, free T-shirts, and free water bottles.

BlueCare relies heavily on member input in tailoring materials and practices. The organization has established member advisory panels for each region. These panels are made up of BlueCare members, staff, and patient advocates. The panels provide input into educational materials and mailings, enhancing the likelihood that these materials will be used by members at large. To remove any barrier to participation in the member advisory panels, BCBST pays transportation and hotel fees for all participants.

In summary, BCBST, through a massive effort, has built, in-house, the expertise required to take care of vulnerable members of the population. In addition to the satisfaction of providing coordinated care to vulnerable TennCare members within the allotted budget, this effort has benefited the organization as a whole by serving as a laboratory in which new business practices can be tested.

Another organization that has successfully used the carve-in strategy to achieve many of the central ethical obligations for care of vulnerable populations is the University of Pittsburgh Medical Center (UPMC) Health Plan. UPMC Health Plan is a much younger organization than BCBST, and its programs with respect to vulnerable members of the population are not nearly as extensive. UPMC Health Plan, therefore, illustrates an earlier phase of evolution toward caring for vulnerable members of the population.

UPMC Health Plan's actions with respect to vulnerable members of the population have largely been taken to meet the requirements of state mandates. The state of Pennsylvania directs insurers to address the special needs of members of vulnerable populations. This is accomplished through two legislative mechanisms: the Department of Public Welfare regulates what must be provided for those on Medical Assistance, and *Pennsylvania Act 68* provides regulations for HMOs. The Public Welfare rules are extensive and specific: HMOs are required to provide members the opportunity to communicate in the member's first language, provide transportation to and from appointments, provide early and periodic screening and diagnostic tests (EPSDTs) for pediatric patients, and provide targeted case management for members with HIV. HMOs are also required to create special needs units to address the social and other needs of vulnerable patients that may affect their health, conduct outreach to vulnerable populations, and establish a 24-hour-a-day hotline to assist members in their interactions with the HMO.[1]

Pennsylvania Act 68, meant to apply to all HMOs operating in the state, adds to this list of requirements: Care must be available to members within a specified distance from their homes, comprehensible written materials describing benefits must be provided, and a plan must be filed as to how the HMO will meet the needs of people with physical disabilities.[2]

All these state regulations, despite their requirements for several specific care programs, are still general enough to allow room for significant variation in how HMOs in the state comply with their broader mandates. UPMC Health Plan has sought explicitly to fulfill the spirit of the mandates to ensure the provision of high-quality care to the most vulnerable patients in the population.

To meet these requirements and best serve the needs of its vulnerable members, UPMC Health Plan attempts to perform a thorough needs assessment of all new Medical Assistance (MA) members. All new MA members are interviewed individually and asked to complete a Health Risk Assessment Tool. Member/provider service representatives phone new members and inquire whether the members need assistance with housing, employment, child care, transportation, job training, access to sufficient, affordable food, or to schools for their children. If the members have identifiable needs unrelated to health care, they are referred to community service organizations in their area. During this contact, new members are also apprised of the services available to them: regular check-ups, preventive care, diagnostic care, and health education.

Based on the initial interview and the Health Risk Assessment Tool, members with special needs are identified and assigned to the special needs unit. The special needs unit consists of trained nurses, social workers, and other staff members. They supply home nursing visits, home health aide visits, homemaker services, nutritional consultations, nutritional supplements, and some medical supplies not covered by Medical Assistance to MA members with HIV/AIDS. The special needs unit also works with pregnant women to make sure they receive prenatal care.

One function of the special needs unit is to develop relationships with the community and identify community resources that will improve members' lives. These resources are not necessarily directly related to health-care benefits, but they may contribute indirectly to improving health status. The special needs unit looks at the impact of the community on members' lives, and the staff work to identify and fill gaps in the community service network.

To fulfill its mission, the special needs unit has found it necessary at times to "stretch" the medical benefit. Stretching the benefit means seeking answers that lie beyond stipulated limits on coverage when it is necessary to help a patient. We were told the story of one patient whose needs led the special needs unit to take this approach. The patient was a single mother of three children on MA. One of the children had severe asthma and required treatments with a nebulizer. The standard single nebulizer provided under the benefit was large, heavy, and difficult to transport. The mother, however, had to take her children by bus to a day care center that was across town from their home before she went to work each day. Frequently, she would forget to bring the nebulizer. If the asthmatic child began to wheeze, the mother would be called at work; she would have to leave work, go home, get the nebulizer, and bring it to the day care center. She was missing work on a regular basis, and the child was still having frequent asthma attacks that required medical attention. The special needs caseworker recognized that this family needed a second nebulizer, but knew it wouldn't be covered under the terms of the benefit package. The caseworker located a company that refurbishes nebulizers and got it to agree to donate a secondhand device to the family. She herself brought the nebulizer to the day care center so the mother would not have to bring the one from home every day. The intervention improved the child's health and decreased the frequency of the mother's absences from her job.

Building Excellence in "Carved-Out" Care
for Vulnerable Populations

Harvard Pilgrim Health Care (HPHC), in contrast to BCBST and UPMC Health Plan, chose to "carve out" its care for vulnerable populations. HPHC has a longstanding organizational commitment to serving vulnerable members of the population. This commitment dates back to one of its predecessor organizations, Harvard Community Health Plan. HPHC's organizational mission statement includes the goals of bringing "care within the reach of as many people as possible" and of supporting "our clinical staff members in teaching, clinical research, and community activities, including those that aim to aim to reduce suffering among the most needy members of society."

HPHC's commitment to the vulnerable members of the community is visible in its longstanding care of the Medicaid population. Ultimately, as HPHC grew beyond its original core staff-model structure into a mixed-model HMO, it chose to carve out the care for the Medicaid population in order to partner with an organization that had extensive experience managing the care of Medicaid patients through an extended network. Prompting this decision was the reality that HPHC was having increasing difficulty managing the costs of caring for its Medicaid population, with losses of $5–$7 million per year. HPHC was deeply committed to the care of the full spectrum of patients in the community, but it did not have the resources to cross-subsidize this level of ongoing losses. HPHC also had to admit that it lacked the internal expertise for managing care in this population across a broad network of providers. The solution was to find a long-term partner to help manage the care of the Medicaid population.

HPHC didn't have to look far. It contracted with Neighborhood Health Plan (NHP), a Massachusetts-based organization that had gained national recognition for its expertise in improving the care of the most challenging vulnerable patients in the Medicaid population. The business plan for the partnership between HPHC and NHP made it clear that HPHC expected to continue to experience financial losses on the Medicaid line of business. However, the mission of serving the whole community, particularly the most needy, was deemed important enough that HPHC elected to accept financial losses, provided they could be maintained at a low enough level that the organization as a whole was not jeopardized.

The care program of NHP that HPHC envied most is worth closer examination. NHP had developed a unique model of care with excellent results for two distinct vulnerable patient populations: patients with advanced AIDS and patients with severe disability. The program, called the Community Medical Alliance (CMA), is a clinical care system contracting with the Massachusetts Medicaid Program on a fully capitated basis to pay for and deliver a comprehensive set of benefits to these patients. Both populations traditionally have exceedingly high health-care costs and suffer from fragmented, uncoordinated care. The CMA program has successfully lowered the costs of caring for these patients while simultaneously improving the quality of services and increasing patient satisfaction.

CMA combines several unique features in its model of care. Working with the state of Massachusetts, CMA pioneered the use of health-status-adjusted premiums to support the creation of improved delivery systems for its target populations. Derived from past fee-for-service costs, the capitated rates for these extremely complex patients provide the financial resources to drive innovation in care management. Over time, it was shown that CMA could take premiums lower than average fee-for-service costs for these patients and create new systems of care that improved health-care coordination and outcomes. And CMA could do this while making a sustainable organizational profit. This was a classic "win-win" example of the potential of good managed care.

In the programs developed by CMA, care is provided to each enrollee through a primary care physician, teamed with a trained nurse-practitioner. This team is empowered with complete authority to admit patients for hospital care, refer them to specialists, or otherwise allocate resources from a wide network of home and community services with one phone call and without risk of financial penalty or loss. CMA focuses heavily on prevention and early intervention strategies to reduce secondary complications in its patient population, reasoning that funding systematic, rapid, in-home, personalized responses will reduce overall hospital and specialty costs. The program promotes education and self-management strategies for its patients and focuses on social support and mental health services as an essential part of the solution to finding alternatives to hospital use and expenditures. CMA provides specialized foster care, rapid-response crisis intervention services in lieu of emergency room or psychiatric care, private-duty nursing, transportation, day treatment, and drug detoxification services on demand. These elements of the care program were created with significant input from the affected patient populations and their advocates.

Results from CMA are impressive. Enrollee satisfaction has been consistently high. The program has also documented a high degree of achievement of defined markers for quality of care. For example, patients with advanced HIV and concomitant drug use have had their rates of adherence with highly active antiretroviral treatment (HAART) regimens go from essentially zero to over 50%. It is clear that CMA has saved many lives among this population. And CMA has accomplished these improvements while keeping total health-care costs significantly below the cost baseline of the previous fee-for-service system. Much of the savings are attributable to greatly reduced use of the hospital. CMA does not scrimp on costs for other services and attributes its success to allocation of a "considerable percentage of the capitation payments to fund home health, durable medical equipment, primary care, and mental health services as alternatives to hospital care" (Master, 1998).

Linking to Community Public Health Resources

Health Net is a for-profit insurer, based in California, with a great deal of experience and expertise in caring for members of vulnerable populations. The health plan has participated in Medicaid (Medi-Cal) for over 15 years and has approximately 500,000 Medicaid enrollees all over the state. Health Net's level of commitment to the care of vulnerable populations runs deep, and through its long experience managing the care of large numbers of Medicaid patients, the organization has developed many exemplary programs. We will describe some of these, but will focus on the plan's distinctive strategy of partnering with the community public health sector to devise coordinated approaches to the care of vulnerable populations.

Health Net has focused a great deal of attention on member services for its Medicaid population. The health plan has a telephone-based member services department that addresses both clinical and administrative issues, so members only have one phone number to remember. This one-stop shopping permits Health Net to track problems. The telephones are staffed 24 hours a day, seven days a week. The sheer scale of Medicaid member services at Health Net is staggering: the department handles approximately 5,000 calls per day. Member services handles all issues: primary care provider changes, coverage denial appeals, problems with identification cards, claims assistance, and triage for medical problems. The call center has a staff that speaks seven languages, and the department utilizes AT&T's language phone line if translation of other languages is needed.

One of the major functions of the member services department is to identify physicians for members. The goal is to preserve existing physician–member relationships and to ensure that members are connected with their physicians promptly in order to assure timely care. Another member services department initiative has been an outgoing call center. New Medicaid members are called 30, 60, and 90 days after enrollment. The purpose of these calls is to welcome new members, identify those in need of outpatient medical care, and find out why members disenroll. Health Net successfully contacts approximately 25% of its new enrollees.

Two other important exemplary aspects of Health Net's care for vulnerable populations have evolved from California state mandates: needs assessments and community advisory committees. The state of California mandates that managed care organizations perform needs assessments for the counties they serve. Health Net has completed assessments in four counties by surveying community-based organizations to assess their needs for health education and by identifying and interviewing key health informants, such as community and religious leaders, about their views on health. The surveys have yielded several important findings: vulnerable patients do not understand the managed care system; they are concerned that providers are not culturally and linguistically sensitive; they have to travel too far to attend health programs; and they have a great need for health programs in areas such as smoking cessation, childhood asthma, teen pregnancy, and prenatal care. Health Net's response has been to develop interventions to address each of these barriers to good care. The health plan is developing a cultural competency training program for providers; educational materials are being prepared in the languages spoken by a significant proportion of the population; telephone-based smoking cessation and lactation programs have been introduced; and some health education programs are being instituted in Head Start centers, a place where mothers spend time with their children.

Health Net's second important initiative in response to a state mandate is the establishment of its community advisory committees (CACs). While the existence of such committees is mandated by the state, Health Net has taken this concept well beyond the minimum legal requirement. The CACs are a mechanism whereby vulnerable members can have a voice in their health care. The CACs offer reactions to culturally appropriate materials, establish education and outreach priorities, and provide input for community needs assessments. Members of the CACs include representatives from community-based organizations as well as consumers, advocates, and representatives from local public health programs. Health Net found that, in order to recruit CAC participants who reflected the Medicaid patient base, it had to provide transportation to CAC meetings, child care during the meetings, and a stipend for participants. One of the first projects Health Net initiated, based on CAC input, was the creation of a childhood asthma video for parents, which was dubbed into multiple languages. The CACs were directly involved in script revisions and in the development of a "peak flow diary." The video has been so successful that it is being shared with members from other managed care organizations.

Notwithstanding the exemplary programs described above, the most innovative aspect of Health Net's approach to vulnerable populations is its department of public health services (DPHS). While the state mandates that all plans develop a memorandum of understanding for carving out public health functions, Health Net has gone far beyond simply creating such a document. In 1997, Health Net created the DPHS to manage the broad range of areas of interface between the health plan and the county and state public health system. Creating the DPHS was intended to improve outcomes for members, eliminate service denials, maximize usage of public health resources, and provide seamless health care to members of vulnerable populations. But the overriding vision was that Health Net, as a health plan, had an integral role to play in partnering with the public health system to improve the care of vulnerable patients.

The staff of the DPHS includes six people who have master's degrees in public-health-related fields; many of the staff members have worked in the past for a county health department, so they are familiar with the public system and committed to serving this underserved population. Among its initiatives, the DPHS has implemented a strategic plan to encourage breast-feeding, created tuberculosis contracts with county health departments to ensure full treatment, and established a Hepatitis A program for schools. Members of the DPHS, as well as other Health Net employees, participate in public health advisory boards to develop statewide programs and policies. From its beginnings in 1997, the DPHS has come to symbolize the potential for coordinated action between managed care and public health. Health Net's experience has shown that this partnership can have significant benefits for the care of vulnerable populations and for the health of entire communities.

Ensuring Access for All

Group Health Cooperative of Puget Sound (Group Health) has created yet another distinctive approach to caring for vulnerable patients, one that is not emulated by many other health plans. An essential aspect of the Group Health mission is to provide care within the community to the greatest number possible. Group Health has interpreted this mission as extending its responsibilities beyond its own members to those vulnerable patients in the community who lack health insurance. Through direct provision of care to patients without insurance, and through a subsidy program for uninsured and underinsured individuals, Group Health seeks to ensure access for all.

The most distinctive elements of Group Health's care of vulnerable populations are administered through two programs: dues grants and the charity care program. (Recently, these two programs were administratively merged into a sponsored care department, but their objectives and methods have remained the same.) These programs are targeted to increase access to care for individuals and families without health insurance and with incomes below 200% of the poverty level. They also serve as a bridge for patients who are at risk of losing their health insurance before they can get new employer coverage or apply for public programs. The dues grant program waives current enrollees' Group Health premiums for six months during times of hardship. The charity care program waives fees for emergency services provided to poor, uninsured patients at Group Health clinics and hospitals. Charity care provides complete coverage for care in the emergency room as well as access to follow-up care for 30 days following the initial visit. Group Health has endeavored to make enrollment in these programs as easy as possible.

Despite the altruistic flavor of these two programs, Group Health also sees a business argument for their approach to the care of vulnerable populations. For one thing, the charity care program keeps Group Health from wasting time and effort pursuing bad debt. The dues grant program has fostered tremendous enrollee loyalty. But the business arguments are not what led to the inspiration for these programs. In 2000 they cost Group Health in excess of $700,000, and no cost-benefit analysis could justify the business argument for continued investment at this level. Group Health's history and culture as an organization, however, have positioned it to view its role as something more than a service organization to its enrollees. Its mission is to extend the benefits of coordinated health care to the entire community. In the face of the U.S. health-care system's failure to provide universal access to care, Group Health takes an activist stance and maintains a broad conception of its role in caring for vulnerable patients. This consistency of vision between its organizational ethics, its care of vulnerable populations, and its approach to community benefits is a theme we will pick up again in the next chapter.

LESSONS LEARNED

Although the various organizational approaches discussed in this chapter differ in their specifics, all share an underlying ethical commitment to providing high-quality care for vulnerable members of the population. These organizations feel that they exist to do much more than manage the insurance risk of their enrollees; they are there to manage care with compassion and foresight and with a sophistication that allows them to care well for even the most vulnerable of patients while competing successfully in the market. For the medical directors of these organizations, it was often a passion for improving the care of vulnerable populations that led them into managed care organizations in the first place. And each has found that passion supported by the culture, mission, and everyday ethical decision making of his or her organization.

Despite the differing competitive strains and the unique elements that mark the distinctive outlines of these organizations' approaches, we can find common ground among many of the exemplary aspects of the specific care programs.

Making Contact

Many vulnerable individuals are members of groups that have been relatively disenfranchised in society. When they first join a health plan, there is often an initial psychological barrier to making contact with the insurer since these individuals may be intimidated by large, established organizations, and experience has taught them not to expect to receive personal attention and satisfaction when they have a problem. BCBST, UPMC Health Plan, and Health Net have all addressed this initial barrier by phoning new members to demonstrate a personal connection and to teach them how to get the help they need to navigate the healthcare system effectively. These organizations have also tried to make themselves less intimidating to all members on an ongoing basis by simplifying the process for members to contact them. Single 1-800 numbers for all questions and answers is an example of a simple yet meaningful organizational response to the plight of vulnerable members.

Connecting to the Community

While vulnerable groups may distrust large organizations, they generally have strong relationships and support structures within their own communities. All of the exemplary programs we evaluated have been able to form strong alliances with these trusted "resources" already in the communities. It hasn't always been easy or quick, but health plans have worked hard to build relationships with existing community organizations and community leaders. These leaders can then act as a bridge between the health care organizations and vulnerable members.

Focusing on Access

Ensuring access to appropriate care at the appropriate time is an absolutely central focus of exemplary programs that care for vulnerable populations. Vulnerable patients often face inherent barriers to getting treatment, be it a lack of insurance, the inability to speak English, a difficult social situation, or the nature and severity of their illness. Exemplary care programs for these patients must therefore focus their attention on a broad definition of access to care. We saw organizations with years of experience that knew just how difficult it could be to help vulnerable patients get the care they need. These organizations had developed multifaceted approaches to improve the access of their vulnerable members. All organizations strove to minimize the distance members needed to travel to obtain clinical services. Each organization also had systems in place to locate providers of the same ethnic or linguistic background for new patients; all provided translation services in clinical as well as administrative settings, transportation to and from appointments for some segments of the population, and child care services in some settings. Whereas some of these features were mandated by state legislation, exemplary practices stood out because of their broad integration of all these approaches within a constant, never-flagging focus on improving access to care.

Assessing Health Needs

One of the hallmarks of vulnerable populations is that they have many and varied health needs, often related to the social and economic determinants of health. As health-care organizations strive to serve this population effectively, many have found that vigorously assessing and addressing these needs, even those beyond the usual definition of medical services, produces better health outcomes, often in a more cost-efficient manner. As we saw in this chapter, organizations such as BCBST and Health Net have formal structures, such as member advisory committees, through which they can learn from vulnerable members themselves what they feel the health priorities are in the community and what they need from the organization to meet these broad health needs. UPMC Health Plan has focused its efforts on needs assessments of individual members, contacting them at home to ask them about their care and their situation at home and at work and to develop a plan to address their most pressing needs. And the CMA program, nested within

HPHC through its partnership with Neighborhood Health Plan, is entirely predicated on changing the focus of health care from the delivery of medical services to a global and comprehensive plan to address the causes of illness and disability in vulnerable populations.

Assessing and acting upon the broad health needs of vulnerable populations reflects a deep understanding of the social determinants of health. It represents the best of what the public health perspective has to offer to organized medicine. Our field studies demonstrate that health-care organizations in competitive markets, seeking to use limited resources wisely and to succeed financially, can benefit enormously from concerted efforts to integrate this vision of health into their systems of care for vulnerable populations. The opportunity to learn from the experience and expertise of programs such as those discussed in this chapter should encourage other organizations to hold on to their value of caring for the neediest members of society. It can be done.

NOTES

1. "Pennsylvania Department of Public Works Office of Medical Assistance Programs RFP" is available at <http://www.dpw.state.pa.us/omap/rfp/omaprfp.asp>. Accessed on May 2, 2002.

2. "Pennsylvania Health Law Project's Analysis of Act 68" is available at <http://www/libertyresources.org/mc/mc-co-8.html>. Accessed on May 2, 2002.

7

COMMUNITY BENEFITS

A development officer at the Metropolitan Museum of Art in New York City calls the chief executive of a national health plan to ask whether the company would be willing to spend $50,000 to be a "platinum" sponsor of an upcoming art show. The show focuses on nineteenth century American art and will be open for three months. Other confirmed major sponsors include a large bank headquartered in New York and an airline. For top-tier sponsorship, the health plan will be listed with the two other major sponsors on advertising for the show and will be able to host at least one private reception and showing of the exhibit. The CEO pauses. He lives in New York and believes strongly in the value of the arts, yet he also knows that his senior medical director has been asked to make budget cuts in free immunization and health fair programs that the company has supported in the past. Should the health plan sponsor the art show if it means cutting back further on its health-related activities? Maybe the health plan can do both, although the CEO worries about the pressure he is under from Wall Street analysts to trim administrative costs. And, after all, the health plan does pay taxes and has always provided good jobs with excellent benefits. Does being a good corporate citizen require it to do yet more for the community?

The CEO of a regional nonprofit health plan checks her appointment list and sees that she is to meet today with the executive director of her health plan's foundation. The foundation is the entity through which the health plan contributes to the community, but in recent years, operating losses have forced the plan to cut back severely on this line item of its budget. Now the tide has finally turned. The health plan is back in the black, and its operating surpluses are accumulating. That's the good news. The bad news, at least from the CEO's viewpoint, is that she is now swamped with hundreds of good proposals for what to do with the extra money available. Higher provider payments, new disease management programs, staff retention bonuses, information systems upgrades; requests for all these and more are on her desk. The foundation's executive director has proposed that the health plan double his budget and, to prevent wide swings in the future, he wants budgets for the foundation to be set formally as an unchangeable percent of corporate revenue. The CEO takes a deep breath and wonders how to balance this request against all the other needs of the organization she is being asked to respond to.

The idea that large health care organizations bear some responsibility for contributing to the general welfare of the community is not new. Legally, it dates to the Internal Revenue Service (IRS)'s criteria for granting hospitals a tax-exempt status. But with the growth in the role of for-profit organizations, increased vertical integration to provide more comprehensive health services, and consolidation in what had traditionally been a local industry, there has been growing interest in trying to define and quantify more precisely what an appropriate community benefit should be (Schlesinger et al., 1998). Some executives of for-profit health care organizations have expressed skepticism that they have a responsibility to contribute to the community; they point out that they, unlike their nonprofit competitors, pay taxes into the public coffers. It is not fair in a competitive system to ask them to contribute further to the community (Hasan, 1996). However, many for-profit, as well as nonprofit, organizations do view community benefits as part of their corporate responsibility. But how much should each organization pay to fulfill its obligation to the community? And what type of community benefits should be expected from health-care organizations? Free care? Health education? Sponsorship of local sports teams and the public arts? These questions frame the ethical and practical questions facing health-care organizations that made community benefits one of the ethical domains of the BEST project.

BACKGROUND

We define community benefits as those services and resources of a health-care organization that are used primarily for the benefit of individuals or groups who are not members of the plan itself. The defining element of community benefits is that they are primarily directed outside the plan, its employees, staff, and premium-paying members. Precisely what those benefits are and the overarching vision they fit into are ethical decisions.

The competing ethical values in decisions regarding community benefits can be summarized in two polar views. In a widely noted editorial in the *New England Journal of Medicine*, health-care executive Malik Hasan, M.D, expressed one of these views by arguing that the only two obligations of for-profit health plans are to provide top-quality health care to their members and well-paying, satisfying jobs to their employees (Hasan, 1996). Hasan cast doubt on the putative community benefits provided by nonprofit health plans, claiming that these benefits are often superficial, hardly holding a candle to the community benefit generated by the taxation of for-profit organizations. Diverting financial resources to sponsor cultural events, provide medications, or offer charity care limits managed care's ability to provide members the health care they paid for and need. According to Hasan, a health plan that pays its fair share of taxes and uses its financial and human resources to ensure that every member receives the best available care is amply fulfilling its social responsibility. So-called community benefits seem morally attractive, but really obscure the harm that is done to members by depriving them of the full measure of health care they have paid for and rightfully expect.

The contrary view holds that community benefits are an integral part of the ethical obligation of all health care organizations for several distinct reasons (Nudelman and Andrews, 1996; Schlesinger and Gray, 1998). First, there is a long tradition of health-care institutions providing community benefits. Many hospitals were originally set up as charitable institutions to minister to the poor. And over the decades, American hospitals have frequently and routinely provided free care to the uninsured. In addition, they have provided other services to neighboring communities, such as targeting jobs to local residents or providing free immunizations. Indeed, in some cases, this community benefit has gone from being a purely voluntary effort to being codified, with state laws requiring nonprofit hospitals and other health-care facilities to have documented plans for community benefits. Some states, such as California and Massachusetts, have extended the requirements for documentation of community benefits to managed care organizations as well. Massachusetts has delineated nine principles to guide HMOs in developing their community benefits program (see Table 7–1). Importantly, the justification for these principles is based on the need of HMOs licensed in Massachusetts to help "meet the growing and pressing health care needs of underserved and uninsured populations" (Attorney General, Commonwealth of Massachusetts, 2000). Nothing in this justification would seem to exempt for-profit health-care organizations from an equal responsibility.

Finally, it is argued that being a good corporate citizen by providing charitable contributions directly to the neighboring community is a fundamental American obligation of all businesses, whether they be in health care or not. According to this view, while enhancing profits and increasing stockholder wealth are central goals of for-profit corporations, so too are strengthening and enriching the local communities in which they operate. Many corporations have created charitable foundations to funnel resources back to the community. Airlines, oil companies, car companies, and telephone carriers routinely sponsor cultural, educational, and related activities. Why then shouldn't the same be expected of health-care organizations? In fact, outside of the managed care system, other health-care companies in the United States routinely allocate funds for community benefit programs. For example, many pharmaceutical companies have created charitable foundations, while others sponsor a variety of cultural and educational programs. Indeed, one of the largest charitable foundations in the United States is that of a health-care company, Eli Lilly.

The notion that the community benefits provided by for-profit companies should be restricted to paying taxes and providing employment thus seems contrary to the tradition of major American corporations. It is also at variance with legal precedents. In a famous 1953 court case, *A.P. Smith Mfg. Co.* vs. *Barlow*,[1] the New

Table 7–1. Massachusetts's HMO community benefits principles

---

1. The governing body of each HMO should adopt and make public a Community Benefits Policy Statement setting forth its commitment to a formal Community Benefits Program.
2. The governing body and senior management of the HMO should be responsible for overseeing the development and implementation of the Community Benefits Program, the resources to be allocated, and the administrative mechanisms for the regular evaluation of the Program.
3. The governing body and senior management of the HMO should seek assistance and participation from HMO members and the community in developing and implementing the HMO's Community Benefits Program, and in defining the targeted population and the specific health care needs to be addressed by the Community Benefits Program.
4. Each HMO should develop its Community Benefits Program based upon an assessment of the health care needs and resources of the identified populations, particularly lower- and moderate-income communities. The Program should consider the health care needs of a broad spectrum of age groups and health conditions.
5. The HMO should develop and market products which would attract all segments of the population.
6. The HMO should strive to offer and promote, consistent with existing laws and regulations, direct enrollment for nongroup coverage and continue to work toward insurance market reform so that managed care will be an option for all working families and individuals.
7. The HMO should take steps to reduce cultural, linguistic, and physical barriers to accessible health care at key points of patient contact.
8. The HMO should strive to help Massachusetts consumers who are about to lose coverage or who are uninsured, to maintain or obtain, as applicable, health care coverage, at least for limited periods of time, at reduced or subsidized rates.
9. The HMO should make an Annual Community Benefits Report available upon request to the public at the HMO and through the headquarters of the Massachusetts Association of HMOs (MAHMO), where the Report will also be available upon request to the public and to the Office of the Attorney General. The Report should describe the HMO's level of community benefits expenditures and describe the HMO's approach to establishing those expenditures.

Jersey Supreme Court ruled that the corporation could legally make charitable contributions. A major effect of this ruling was to create legal permission for many types of corporate charitable contributions, leaving it up to corporations to decide whether to make them or not. The New Jersey court seemed, however, to argue that there was an implied obligation for corporations to contribute resources beyond general taxes to the community: "[M]odern conditions require that corporations acknowledge and discharge social as well as private responsibilities as members of the communities within which they operate." The ruling granting permission for corporations to make charitable contributions was subsequently codified in the corporation laws in many states, giving all corporations the power to "make donation for the public welfare or for charitable, scientific, or educational purposes."[2] Indeed, the California and New York corporation laws make clear that donations need not just be for "corporate objectives" but can be made "regardless of specific corporate benefit for the public welfare or for community fund, hospital, charitable, education, scientific, civic, or similar purposes."[3] This is a view shared by the IRS; federal tax law permits corporations to make charitable contributions without limiting these contributions to business purposes.

Despite the arguments proposed by Hasan and others, therefore, the weight of ethical thinking, corporate tradition, and legal precedent supports the notion of corporate responsibility for contributions to the community. And, in fact, most health-care organizations, whether for-profit or nonprofit, do dedicate at least some resources to community benefit. Several important ethical questions remain, however. An obvious first consideration is how much is enough? How much money is appropriate to dedicate to community benefits? One percent of gross revenue? Ten percent of net income? Does it matter if the health plan is making or losing money overall? Does it matter how much money is being allocated for community benefit by competitors in the marketplace? In the tough economic cycle for health plans in the United States in the late 1990s, many plans faced difficult questions about whether they should fund community benefits as a set percentage of revenue or as a discretionary line-item expenditure that might vary, based on the financial performance of the health plan. Clearly, these options reflect different views about how integral community benefits are to the mission of the health plan.

A second issue revolves around what *type* of community benefits should be provided. Should they be restricted to health-care benefits or include non-health-care activities? Some might argue that, as health-care companies, health plans should focus on improving community health. The fragmented U.S. health-care system presents ample opportunity for health plans and other health-care organizations to help provide care to the uninsured and underinsured patients in every community. We have seen in the last chapter an example of just such an approach at Group Health. There are also opportunities to support community health through health education, violence prevention, and other similar programs. Another view contends, however, that such health-related activities can be surreptitiously co-opted by the business goals of a health-care company and that community benefits should therefore focus on non-health-related activities, such as support of the arts or education. According to this view, the only way for community benefits to reflect a commitment to the community free of any self-serving interests is for them to target needs unrelated to health care. As an example, until very recently, the Eli Lilly Foundation expressed just this sentiment through an explicit policy of not funding health-related activities.

Once it is decided what type of community benefits will be given, there are still further questions about how to determine what specific projects should be funded and how to evaluate whether the community benefits are really beneficial. While determining the process for establishing funding priorities may seem like an operational issue, it necessarily involves key value choices. For instance, deciding to involve the community in determining funding priorities affirms the important value of community empowerment. Similarly, if it is determined that health care will be the focus of community benefits, who, what, and where will be the focus? Will the money go to children or the homeless or the poor? Or only to poor, homeless children? Should the money go toward prevention, primary care, or the improvement of care for patients with rare diseases? These choices can only be made by prioritizing key ethical values.

ETHICAL VALUES AND CENTRAL ETHICAL OBLIGATIONS

Each of these choices—whether to provide community benefits, how much to provide, what type to provide, and how to prioritize targets within a particular type of benefit—involves the balancing or integration of competing values held by any health-care organization in a competitive market. These competing values are nearly identical to those that come into play in decisions regarding the care of vulnerable populations: on one side, the altruistic values of commitment to community and the desire to invest in improving the health of all its members, and on the other, the values of stewardship of limited resources and the drive to ensure the economic success of the organization.

We have identified two central ethical obligations to guide health-care organizations as they manage this ethical tension (see Table 7–2). The first obligation is to recognize explicitly a commitment to communal solidarity. The community with which a health-care organization expresses solidarity can be defined by geography, health status, ethnicity, or socioeconomic background. Thus, the community does not have to be narrowly defined, and it is perfectly possible for a national health plan to identify a community or set of communities for which it establishes a special commitment. Broader definitions of community are, in fact, necessary for a true sense of solidarity to emerge. The concept of solidarity, as discussed in the previous chapter, includes an affective component that extends the organization's commitment beyond the dispassionate claims of justice. Solidarity combines the concepts of fraternity and mutuality to connote a collective obligation and mutual

Table 7–2. Central ethical obligations for community benefit

EXEMPLARY ETHICAL ORGANIZATIONS MUST:
1. Demonstrate communal solidarity.
2. Continually seek community empowerment.

reciprocity based on feelings of social unity (Wildt, 1999). As an ethical obligation, solidarity counterbalances what many see as the overemphasis in American culture on individuality and the values of capitalism. It is a key characteristic of health-care organizations with exemplary community benefit programs.

The second central ethical obligation is community empowerment. Just as empowerment of its own consumers means that a health-care organization must give them opportunities to make their own choices and shape their own destinies, empowerment of communities requires that organizations do the same for them by developing ways to seek out their ideas, involve them in deliberation and decision making, and offer them the chance to determine priorities among the issues and programs that affect them.

Even among community benefit programs guided by these two central ethical obligations, operational methods can differ considerably. In the next section we describe several distinctive programs that demonstrate the diversity of exemplary ethical approaches to realizing communal solidarity and empowerment in community benefits.

EXEMPLARY PRACTICES

Community Benefits as Corporate Culture

The Group Health Cooperative of Puget Sound (Group Health) has an extensive commitment to community benefits that ranges from support of research and teaching to assisting the uninsured and supporting initiatives to improve the quality of care at community health sites. Over the years, Group Health has had to confront many critical decisions about community benefits: How should these benefits align with the organization's strategic plan? Should there be one focus or a variety of priorities? What level of financial support should be devoted to community benefits during periods of financial losses for the organization? Throughout the organization's history, its culture has provided a consistent foundation for the answers to these questions.

In the previous chapter we described Group Health's exemplary programs to support uninsured patients and disadvantaged enrollees facing an interruption in health-care coverage. Because these programs for the care of vulnerable populations extend beyond Group Health's own membership to include general members of the community, they form an important part of Group Health's community benefit. But there are other elements of Group Health's approach to community benefits that, taken together, demonstrate the consistency and alignment of the entire corporate culture with communal solidarity and empowerment.

At the heart of Group Health's community benefit is the Group Health Foundation. The foundation is structured as a separate 501c(3) corporation with its own board of directors. Begun in 1983 to promote philanthropy and community projects, the foundation receives core operating funding and much of its ancillary services, such as legal services, from Group Health. The foundation also raises money from individuals, foundations, and corporations to fund a variety of grants and programs supporting research, health promotion, and quality of care. Since 1983 it has awarded over 237 grants totaling $3.2 million.

Foundation leaders see several major issues confronting the mission of their organization. One is the challenge of interpreting its community benefit as the geographical reach of the health plan shifts dramatically. In dynamic marketplaces, the defined population of a managed care organization is likely to expand or contract, creating significant barriers to a coherent sense of communal solidarity. This challenge has been particularly acute for Group Health and its foundation because of the long historical link of the health plan to a very specific geographic region. Group Health originated and prospered for decades in the Seattle area, but recently, it has expanded throughout the state of Washington and now has a significant proportion of its membership outside the Puget Sound region. Historically, most of the charitable work of the foundation has been centered in Seattle. This tradition can give the impression that Group Health and the foundation care less about the needs of rural communities in eastern or southern Washington state. In response, the foundation has opened offices in Tacoma and Spokane and has consciously searched for projects to fund outside of Seattle.

A second issue confronting the foundation relates to focus. Instead of being proactive and defining its own charitable priorities, the foundation has, until very recently, waited passively for submitted proposals, resulting in a lack of synergy between funded programs and a diminution of the cumulative impact of the foundation's efforts. In 2000, however, the foundation's board of directors approved a new strategic focus to address this concern. Approximately 75% of the community grantmaking has now been directed toward programs for healthy children and teens, while the remaining grants fund emergent needs that may fall outside this focus.

A third challenge facing the foundation is the need to justify the costs of supporting its activities to Group Health executives and directors. This became an acute problem in the mid-to-late 1990s when Group Health was losing tens of millions of dollars annually and almost went out of business. The approach taken by the foundation's directors in justifying its expense has been multifaceted. Their argument begins with a direct claim that community benefit programs are not just altruism but a key strategic asset. The work of the foundation builds a broader base of trust in the community for Group Health, a trust that proved critical in keeping important accounts and providers on board during the organization's darkest financial days. Communal solidarity, it turns out, is a two-way street. Slash the foundation's budget, and the community's commitment to Group Health will wither and the reason to view Group Health as something special in the marketplace will be extinguished.

The other thrust of the foundation's argument to executives defending the value of its work has centered on the claim that certain health problems, including teen smoking and HIV among drug abusers, cannot be adequately or primarily addressed through the traditional health-care delivery system. These health problems are pernicious and their long-term effects expensive to care for. Only by working with the community through the kind of broad-based programs sustained by the foundation can these problems be addressed. Education and prevention are the tools required to obtain improved health and lower costs in certain high-risk, vulnerable populations. And, the argument concludes, these tools can best be developed through collaborative programs sponsored by the foundation.

As prominent as the foundation is, however, it is not the only mechanism through which Group Health provides community benefits. There are other threads of Group Health's community benefit programs to be found within the health plan itself. The consistency and coordination that Group Health has recently brought to these additional community benefits is another sign of the way that the entire corporate culture of Group Health is aligned with the ethical ideals of community solidarity and empowerment.

Within Group Health itself, prior to 1997, charitable donations and community projects were splintered across different parts of the organization. Over the years, individual initiatives had been supported in a kind of "thousand points of light" approach to charitable contributions. This diffuse approach created great opportunities for individual Group Health employees to design and implement programs to help the community, but it reduced the potential for these programs to find synergy and greater impact through coordination. In addition, the disparate small efforts undermined the visibility and recognition of Group Health's community involvement. One of many illustrative examples of this problem occurred when five different districts within the organization participated in the American Cancer Society's Relay for Life—with no coordination among them. Despite extensive contributions, Group Health fell just $3,000 short of being recognized as a major sponsor of the event—and even failed to recognize what had happened until it was too late to coordinate efforts for the following year.

Consequently, in 1997, Group Health began a new approach. That year, Group Health's new CEO assigned the communications department the task of creating a community relations improvement council to align charitable giving and other community benefits activities with public relations, marketing, and the annual business plan. The membership of the new community relations improvement council came from a cross section of the organization and undertook a systematic approach for coordinating Group Health's internal community benefits initiatives. The council began its work by surveying the public, community leaders, Group Health enrollees, and large employers in the Seattle area to determine what issues were most important to them. In each Group Health district, advisory groups were created to advise the council. These advisory groups were placed directly under the direction of each district manager and medical director, with participation from staff and consumers with interest or expertise in community involvement. The advisory groups were critical elements in Group Health's effort to empower its communities to help establish the principles and priorities that would guide Group Health's community programs.

One important corporate goal for this shift to a more coordinated model was to bring greater cohesion to Group Health's clinical and business priorities. With the input of the advisory groups, Group Health established priorities, including children's health and safety, innovations in prevention, improved access to health information and care for underserved populations, and cultural diversity in health care. These priorities were transmitted simultaneously through the medical and the business branches of Group Health and led to greater collaboration and, ultimately, to much improved alignment of initiatives throughout the organization. For example, children's health became the cover story of the GHC member magazine, the focus of in-clinic posters, and the subject matter for public service announcements with a regional television station. The emphasis on cancer prevention and screening was coordinated through a new in-clinic brochure series and posters, a magazine feature, and through well-organized sponsorship and team involvement in the Komen Foundation's Race for the Cure and in the previous missed-opportunity event: the American Cancer Society's Relay for Life.

Taken as a whole, Group Health's experience with its approach to community benefit programs demonstrates that such programs can flourish, even in competitive markets during hard financial times, as long as an organization has community solidarity and empowerment at the heart of its corporate culture. Furthermore, the coordination of community benefit programs with related initiatives in the clinical and business departments at Group Health has only strengthened the position of those programs within the overall organization. Admittedly, Group Health is a unique organization, even among nonprofit HMOs. Its appreciation for the values of solidarity and empowerment, and its resulting deep connection to the community, have long historical roots. Group Health is a cooperative with consumer governance, born and bred to serve the community from which it sprang. Group Health's culture has remained closely connected to these early roots, and the culture consistently supports measures to sustain community benefits, even during times of financial stress. The Group Health example proves that it is possible, with support throughout nearly every part of the organization, for a health plan, steeped in a tradition of serving the community, to survive and flourish in a competitive market.

Community Benefit Supported by Religious Principle

Holy Cross Health System is a health-care organization consisting of Catholic hospital systems in different regions of the country. The BEST team visited two sites: St. Agnes in Fresno, California, and Mt. Carmel in Columbus, Ohio. At both sites, the community benefit programs seemed virtually endless. The external focus on the community was absolutely pervasive, and unquestioned allegiance to the values of communal solidarity and empowerment permeated every person and every program associated with the organization.

One could not visit Holy Cross's facilities without being struck by the sheer volume of community benefit programs. New programs, old programs, large and small programs—everywhere one looked, there was another benefit program. And every employee of Holy Cross seemed to have working knowledge of all the specific community benefit projects offered by the organization. In the same way that many employees of some organizations are familiar with the corporate mission statement and annual business plans, the employees of Holy Cross all seemed to share the ability to rattle off with pride the long list of their community benefit projects.

While such an extensive community benefits program runs the risk of being diffuse and unfocused, Holy Cross's myriad initiatives are effectively targeted at the very neediest and socially marginal—the poor, minorities, elderly, and children. This focus receives an unchanging source of inspiration from the religious principles underlying Holy Cross's mission. That mission, which we described earlier in our chapter on organizational ethics, bears repeating here as a powerful statement of communal solidarity and empowerment in a competitive health care system:

> Faithful to the spirit of the Congregation of the Sisters of the Holy Cross, the Holy Cross Health System exists to witness Christ's love through excellence in the delivery of health services motivated by respect for those we serve. We foster a climate that empowers those who serve with us while stewarding our human and financial resources.

Further articulating the core values that follow from this mission, Holy Cross includes "respecting every human being," "giving of ourselves in order to respond appropriately to the needs of others" and "through the use of individual and organizational action and influence [enabling] all to participate in society seeking the common good." It is hard to imagine that community benefit programs could find stronger foundations than these.

Because Holy Cross takes community benefit to be integral to its mission, funds for these services are integrated into its regular operating budget and a full business-like accounting of community benefits is performed. Holy Cross Health System aims for each individual facility to provide at least 2% of gross revenues to charity. To evaluate its financial contributions to community benefits, Mt. Carmel has used a Social Accountability Report developed by the Catholic Health Association of American. This report uses generally accepted accounting practices (GAAP) to determine the precise financial contributions to the community. Mt. Carmel's target has been 3% of income allocated to community benefit, and in 1998 this came to over $32 million dollars. Holy Cross feels strongly that adding community benefits to the bottom line in this explicit fashion transmits a powerful message to the executives, financial officers, and employees that these benefits are part of the regular budget, not marginal add-ons. It also makes transparent to the community and state regulators Holy Cross's level of commitment to community benefits.

As noted above, the ethical value of community empowerment is strongly integrated into Holy Cross's mission. The organization follows through on this commitment by performing needs assessments in both a structured and more open-ended manner. On the structured side, in 1995, St. Agnes performed a community survey in Fresno to identify health needs. Fresno, a community with high unemployment, high levels of poverty, and substantial cultural diversity, has a plethora of health needs, but St. Agnes's survey was helpful in identifying the top three priorities: teen pregnancy, substance abuse, and high school dropout rates. In addition, St. Agnes supports Vision 20/20, a new United Way biannual community needs assessment. Similarly, Mt. Carmel works with 22 local churches (not all Catholic) to identify the health needs of their worshippers and help provide care and other programs.

In addition to these structured assessments, Mt. Carmel has a community outreach fund with an open-door policy for proposals from employees and individuals in the community who define their own needs. And sometimes, needs assessment can just happen informally through being sensitive and open. One Holy Cross employee, a vice president for research and development, told us of a trip she took to a small rural town near one of the Holy Cross hospitals. After arriving in the town, she went to a local bar to get a soda. The bar patrons stared at her and then inquired whether she was a "penguin." She said she was not, but added she was certainly interested in finding out what kind of health issues the people in the town were most concerned about. The men asked for education on prostate cancer and screening for heart disease. It was not long before Holy Cross made sure they got it.

We learned in depth of two exemplary programs at St. Agnes dedicated to specific illnesses: sickle-cell disease and AIDS. Initially using tobacco settlement funds, a nurse took the initiative to design and establish a program to care for patients with sickle-cell disease and thalassemia. The nurse educates patients and families about self-care and early intervention for sickle crises. In addition, local physicians are provided case-management and education programs on sickle-cell disease. In order to improve continuity of care, the program has built relationships with a local pediatric hospital that cares for many of the pediatric patients with the disease. Furthermore, the program has worked with the state Department of Corrections to educate and care for prisoners with sickle-cell disease. The newest program initiative is the creation of relationships with academic medical centers to allow for participation in ongoing research on sickle-cell disease. The program has resulted in decreased frequency of emergency room visits, hospital admissions, and decreased average length of stays for sickle-cell patients who do get admitted.

In 1988, St. Agnes began a home-based case-management program for HIV/ AIDS. At the time the program was launched, HIV carried a serious social stigma, yet many young people were coming home to their families to be cared for as they died. The program provides case management in the patient's home as well as skilled nursing care not otherwise covered by insurance. In addition, it provides these patients many other uncovered health-care and social-support services, including dental care, personal attendant services, clothes, and, when desperately needed, furniture and rent. There is no requirement that the patients receive their health care from St. Agnes. Indeed, doctors from Kaiser Permanente regularly refer their local HIV/AIDS patients to the program, although Kaiser provides no financial assistance to it. From the start, the program was continuously and significantly overenrolled. The initial funding provided by the state covered care for only 15 patients a year, but the program actually served 45. Currently, the program cares for 80 clients per month, with 85% of the funding come from the federal government and St. Agnes shouldering the rest.

Another of St. Agnes's community-benefit initiatives is located in Poverello House, a well-established soup kitchen in a poor Fresno neighborhood. Within Poverello House, St. Agnes has created a clinic providing general medical, dental, and some specialty services for its clients and people in the surrounding neighborhood. The clinic is staffed by a full-time nurse practitioner, whose salary is paid for by St. Agnes. In addition, St. Agnes's staff physicians and dentists volunteer their time at the house. St. Agnes provides free medications and instructions on taking them, and offers translation services to people who need them. Across the street from Poverello House is the Holy Cross Center for Women, which provides numerous services, including mental health and medical services, Alcoholics and Narcotics Anonymous meetings, counseling, educational programs in English as a Second Language, computer training, child care during class time, clothing, and baby supplies.

Visiting Poverello House and the Holy Cross Center for Women is a powerful experience. The specific religious inspiration is palpable, but so is an awareness of the atmosphere of safety and empowerment and the depth of the care and caring that spring from common wells of love for one's neighbor. Our final lasting impression was the familiarity of the nurses and staff at Poverello House with the senior St. Agnes executives who were leading us on our tour. The St. Agnes executives had clearly been there often before, by themselves, not to impress VIP visitors, but to touch, help, and serve people in need.

Similar to St. Agnes, Mt. Carmel is located in a poor neighborhood of Columbus, Ohio, and has dedicated significant resources to the disadvantaged. The local churches, including those of many denominations, provide a main mechanism for Mt. Carmel to connect with the community. Mt. Carmel maintains "health stations" at two local non-Catholic churches. These health stations provide nurse and physician services to whoever drops in and seeks care. Hoping to bring them into the health care system, they are especially receptive to African American men. Mt. Carmel also supports health fairs with blood pressure, glucose, and cholesterl screening as well as pneumococcal and flu shots, mammography, educational materials, and referrals for follow-up care. In 1998, Mt. Carmel staffed 14 health fairs that included 658 participants, providing 36 mammograms including 3 referrals for suspicious nodules, 622 cholesterol measurements with 412 elevated levels, and 705 glucose measurements with 76 elevated levels.

Mt. Carmel also uses medical vans to get its services to the local community and to go house-to-house in the neighborhood around the hospital, a poor community, to identify children who have not received their routine immunizations and offer them free shots on the spot. The hospital has also equipped a van that roams the streets of Columbus with regular predetermined stops publicized in the community. The van is staffed by a nurse and physician paid for by Mt. Carmel and is fully equipped, offering laboratory tests, and a wide range of medications typically needed by the homeless who use its services. When appropriate, individuals are referred to the hospital for necessary specialized services.

What are the general lessons from Holy Cross? As with Group Health, the most important lesson may be that when identification with and caring for the community are at the heart of the mission of an organization, the result is a robust program of community benefits. The organizational roots supporting community solidarity and empowerment are different at Holy Cross. They flow from the order's religious history and the strength of its ongoing beliefs. Responding to the needs of others and seeking the common good are core values that have been translated into the stunning breadth and depth of the community programs at Holy Cross.

Religion defines the motivation and the broad focus on those most in need, but it was our impression that this inspiration is broadly conceived and does not lead Holy Cross into an evangelical or paternalistic approach to helping the community. Like Group Health, Holy Cross seeks to reach out into its communities and empower them by listening carefully to their concerns. The agenda and priorities for Holy Cross's community benefits programs come from the communities themselves. Holy Cross is an exemplary example of how to empower the voice of the disadvantaged by first being a good listener.

Focusing Community Benefits on Medical Education and Research

Part of the mission of the Harvard Community Health Plan (HCHP) at its inception in 1969 was to serve "everyone in the community," particularly the "most needy." 1969 was a time when the ideals of community health and social solidarity flourished, and HCHP seemed to embody these ideals, as did Kaiser Permanente, Group Health, and other old staff-model HMOs. As the brainchild of Dr. Robert Ebert, dean of Harvard Medical School, however, HCHP was also born with academic blood in its veins. The health plan mission included a charge to "actively support teaching, research, and community service." By 1980 HCHP had grown to the point where it had decided to create a separate foundation to serve as the main instrument of its community benefits program. The HCHP Foundation's mission was three-fold, and the order in which its components were listed was not accidental: education, research, and community service. Later, in the mid-1990s, HCHP merged with Pilgrim Health Care to become Harvard Pilgrim Health Care (HPHC), and the foundation also changed its name to become the HPHC Foundation. By this time, the foundation was still contributing significantly to teaching and research, but its community service programs had grown significantly and become its dominant priority. However, as financial difficulties engulfed the health plan in the late 1990s, both the funding and the mission of the foundation were subjected to critical reexamination. What emerged was a reorganized community benefits program that adapted to severe budget cuts by emphasizing its commitments to teaching and research while greatly curtailing its community service involvement. How the HPHC Foundation refocused in order to see its legacy survive the near-death experience of its parent organization is a story with important lessons for the community benefits programs of all health-care organizations in competitive markets.

In the early 1990s, the HPHC Foundation's community service program was extensive and varied. Like many other health plan community service programs, it provided financial support for proposals originating from members of the community, but lacked a strong, coherent vision. In the mid-1990s, the primary targets for community projects were made more explicit as part of the agreement with the state to permit the merger of HCHP with Pilgrim Health Care. The agreement mandated spending a minimum of $1.2 million per year on AIDS prevention, violence prevention, health promotion for the elderly, and substance abuse prevention for the homeless. Despite now having a list of priorities, the foundation continued to select programs for funding from the diverse requests and proposals it received from the community. Among the programs the foundation funded were those creating and distributing educational materials for teenagers on AIDS, pregnancy, substance abuse, and violence; exhibits at local museums; home and community interventions on anger management; fitness classes for the elderly; mentoring programs in local high schools; contributions to crisis centers; and support of information resources for the public, such as the Mayor's Health Line and the Massachusetts Poison Control Center. The foundation even allocated resources to be spent on political advocacy at the state level for expanding health coverage for the uninsured. Several of these programs initiated by the foundation received state and national awards for excellence. Funding for community service programs grew each year as they became an ever more central feature of the foundation's efforts.

In 1995 HPHC set its budget for the foundation at $4.5 million per year, significantly more than had been spent on charitable contributions by its two predecessor organizations combined. Approximately $3 million per year was allocated to community service programs; the remaining $1.5 million would go for the support of teaching and research. However, the good times were about to end. In 1999, HPHC announced that it had suddenly discovered it had overall debts in excess of $200 million, and the health plan was put into receivership by the state of Massachusetts while its very survival was in question.

Working in concert with state officials, HPHC's subsequent operating budgets reduced its annual allocation to the foundation by half, to $2.25 million. The foundation was still in control of how to allocate its resources, but with its budget cut in half, it clearly could not continue business as usual. The foundation board had two options. It could reduce support for its programs proportionately across the board, or it could set priorities and use these priorities to guide more selective budget cuts.

The foundation chose to set priorities and, in a reversal of its previous trend, decided that the teaching and research elements of the Foundation's portfolio should receive priority, leaving community service programs to absorb the entire brunt of the budget cuts. Today, only about $625,000 per year is spent for community service programs. Teaching and research, however, continue to receive approximately $1.5 million per year. The decision to prioritize support of teaching and research was a contentious one, but it was guided in part by the hope of saving what was most distinctive about HPHC and its foundation in the marketplace. No other health plan in Massachusetts had a comparable history of engagement in teaching and research. HPHC was the clear leader in integrating teaching and research into its delivery system. Importantly, it had also teamed with Harvard Medical School in 1992 to create the only medical school academic department in the country located in a health plan. These were flagship programs. In the setting of tough decisions requiring draconian measures, the academic roots of HPHC proved deep and lasting.

The entire teaching and research budget of the HPHC Foundation is channeled through a joint HPHC-Harvard Medical School department, the Department of Ambulatory Care and Prevention (DACP). The DACP receives direct support from both HPHC and Harvard Medical School and is thus jointly sponsored. Sitting physically within the health plan, the DACP's faculty have full-fledged academic appointments at Harvard Medical School. Long-range planning and oversight is provided by both sponsoring organizations, symbolized by the fact that the chair of the DACP reports directly to both the dean of Harvard Medical School and the senior medical director of HPHC.

From its inception, the DACP has had an explicit mission to develop educational and research programs for preventive medicine and health care in ambulatory settings. The DACP has grown rapidly over the past decade, and its faculty now includes many nationally recognized experts in primary care and health policy. Most of its operating funds (now over $10 million per year) comes through external grants from sources including the federal government, philanthropic foundations, and private corporations. In addition to its research activities, the DACP exercises the leadership role for Harvard Medical School in developing and managing educational programs for medical students, residents, fellows, and practicing physicians that emphasize primary care, prevention, and clinical epidemiology. The DACP manages all of the clinical precepting and teaching done within HPHC's major affiliated practices, and itself also sponsors several advanced fellowship programs. When the HPHC Foundation decided to cut sharply its community service programs, it was to maintain its core support for one of its acknowledged triumphs: the DACP's unique structure and its mission of population-focused research and teaching.

In one way, the story of HPHC and its foundation provides insight into the fragility of community benefits, even when they are deeply ingrained in the mission of the organization. As originally conceived, community service programs were integral to the activities of the health plan. The language of the mission statement and of various strategic plans made clear that community benefit—including the full trio of community service, education, and research—was fundamental. The wish to serve and benefit the community seems genuine and quite deeply rooted both in the organization's culture and its employees.

But impending death has a way of focusing the mind, and in HPHC's case, the descent into financial chaos led its foundation to refocus its entire approach to community benefits. How does HPHC's choice to prioritize teaching and research relate to the central ethical obligations of communal solidarity and empowerment? The answer is difficult. The sudden financial crisis precluded any attempt to gather broad community input into the decision. From its most central stakeholders, however, HPHC heard that it was worth trying to save the organization *only* if HPHC retained that which it had to offer that was unique. To many, this was HPHC's role as a primary source of connection between academia and the world of managed care. Additionally, a common view was that isolated community benefit initiatives could be revived or started anew if the organization returned to profitability, but it was felt that the teaching and research infrastructure built up over the previous decade could not survive a sudden and deep reduction in its support.

In the end, financial stress made HPHC's commitment to community benefits bend, but not break. And in the reconfigured prioritization of teaching and research over community service programs, it may well be that the HPHC Foundation appropriately chose to go with its strength: the history and tradition of its academic character. Firmly rooting its community benefits within this deeply prized organizational tradition may have been the best way to ensure the ultimate survival of a more robust community benefits program. If economic times do smile once again on HPHC, a broader menu of community service initiatives may be reintroduced and grow. For now, however, there is solace in the fact that HPHC has identified and saved its core commitment. Health-care organizations in competitive markets that face the same trials as HPHC can take heart in this lesson.

A Deep Commitment to the People of Tennessee

There is a single defining characteristic of Blue Cross Blue Shield of Tennessee (BCBST) that provides the inspiration and the framework for all of its community benefit programs: BCBST is a Tennessee company. The company restricts itself to Tennessee; it has repeatedly refused to expand beyond the state into Alabama or Georgia. Being a Tennessee company—in fact and in spirit—explains the source of BCBST's deeply felt communal solidarity with all the people of Tennessee. As their mission statement makes clear:

> Our mission is to provide affordable high quality healthcare benefits and services for all Tennesseans.

Rich, poor; white, black; sophisticated Nashville executives, and illiterate rural farm workers—if you're a Tennessean, BCBST feels a commitment to you and your community. BCBST wants to do whatever it can to provide health coverage to as many Tennesseans as possible. And it wants to do more. As one of the major employers in the state, as a company with a long history of service to the people of Tennessee, and as a graceful grande dame of Tennessee health-care institutions, BCBST takes the notion of being a good corporate citizen seriously. Tom Kinser, the CEO of the company described this view in BCBST's *Caring in the Community: 1998 Community Involvement Report*:

> We are not content just to pay our financial obligations when a subscriber needs health care services. We are committed to the ongoing goal of being a good corporate citizen. And that means caring in the community—working to improve physical, social and emotional concerns.

In the previous chapter, we examined one important manifestation of BCBST's commitment to the Tennessee community: its willingness to take on the challenge of TennCare. Most of BCBST's commercial competitors like Cigna did not join TennCare. But BCBST though it had to do it, that it was obviously the right thing to do, even though the detailed arrangements—financial, political, and otherwise— were far less than optimal and participation might cost BCBST substantial good will among physicians.

BCBST's experiences with the TennCare population has taught the entire company a lot about how to empower and serve any community with significant healthcare needs. The care of vulnerable populations in TennCare provided additional motivation and practical insights that have helped BCBST build excellent statewide community programs aimed at providing education and improving health, with a particular focus on Tennessee's children. The focus on children is pervasive at BCBST, and a variety of interlocking programs have been developed to help disadvantaged children. One is Baby Me Two—a statewide media campaign aimed at increasing women's awareness of the importance of obtaining prenatal care in the first trimester. Another is Shots for Tots, in which BCBST works with county health departments to increase the rate of immunizations among two-year-old children. This program begins with a newborn welcome letter sent to new parents, along with a refrigerator magnet outlining the schedule for immunizations. This is followed up over time with a birthday card sent to parents of one- and two-year-olds that includes a reminder of immunizations that are needed. So far this program has been effective in raising the immunization rates of two-year-old children to 84%, the highest it has ever been in Tennessee.

BCBST also has several programs that target school-aged children. The best known of these is the BC Bear Club for children in kindergarten through third grade. Tennessee has a large population of relatively isolated rural inhabitants who are unlikely to be aware of, or practice, healthy behaviors. Many Tennessee children are at risk of not learning the importance of eating well, exercising, good dental care, not smoking, and other healthy habits. The goal of the BC Bear Club is to educate children (and through them, their parents) and help ingrain healthy habits during their formative years. Children enrolled in the program are given two health education workbooks, stickers, and a membership card. Teachers are provided with special lesson plans. A BC Bear goes to schools to perform an educational skit teaching kids habits such as the importance of brushing their teeth. The program is focused, longitudinal, and uses just about every medium imaginable to get inside the heads of children and start them off with healthy lifestyles. And the BC Bear Club is known to virtually every parent in the state; the program has enrolled over 100,000 children statewide and has 400 participating schools.

BCBST also participates in a wide variety of more traditional corporate community benefit activities. It sponsors the Tennessee Senior Games, an annual event for adults 50 and older, as well as the Eastman 3K fitness walk. It also has been a long-time statewide sponsor of the American Heart Association's Heart Walk, a national walking event that raises money to support research and public education on heart disease. In 1997, the company raised over $70,000 for this event. In addition, BCBST is a sponsor of the Riverbend 5K run that also has a one-mile fun run/walk for families.

Part of BCBST's emphasis on children's health extends to educational needs. When the company upgrades its computers, it donates its older equipment to schools and community organizations. Another education-directed effort is the Adopt-a-School program. BCBST provides financial support to several schools and encourages its employees to volunteer as tutors. Similarly, the company throws back-to-school bashes where school supplies are given to children along with games designed so they can discover health information on their own.

Throughout all these programs flows the unifying theme that BCBST exists to serve the people of Tennessee. That identification is so strong that it even helped determine the corporate response to the question of growth beyond the state borders. The answer: We are a Tennessee company. The clarity of this vision compels BCBST to a deep appreciation for the value of community solidarity. BCBST shows how a geographical self-identification can inspire the development of exemplary programs of community benefits. Although other health-care organizations may not have a map with which they can so neatly define the boundaries of their communities, the success of BCBST may say more about the strength of its community identification than it does about the geographical nature of that identification. BCBST has nurtured a special connection with its broader community— they are all Tennesseans. Group Health and Holy Cross have managed to build different, but nearly equally coherent, visions of the communities with which each organization has a special bond. All health-care organizations should seek to find their own creative ways to reach out and identify communities worth caring about.

LESSONS LEARNED

What additional lessons can be learned from comparing the experience of these diverse examples of community benefits programs? One important common theme is the focus of all the community benefits programs on health and health-care-related activities. The organizations we studied are devoted to ensuring the health of the community; supporting arts, culture, or the environment, no matter how worthy, lacks resonance with the organizations' cultures.

Unlike the products of tire manufacturers, construction companies, or public relations firms, the product of health-care organizations—health—is viewed as special, a key to the American ideal of equal opportunity, and something that should be socially guaranteed. This does not mean that the focus of exemplary community benefit programs should be narrowly construed as providing health-care services. A true commitment to community solidarity expressly broadens the universe of domains relevant to health, including issues of public health and the powerful social determinants of health that are unequally distributed within communities.

We noticed during our investigation that in community benefit programs across the country there was a remarkably consistent emphasis both on illness prevention and on children. This may be a result of the spirit of the times. But it may also reflect the insight that prevention initiatives and children's health are particularly resistant to traditional medical care programs and instead require true community-based interventions to realize improvement. Prevention of complex health problems rarely emerges from a 15-minute doctor's appointment or a quick prescription. The best community benefit programs are steeped in the public health perspectives and techniques that have occupied the fringes of the U.S. health-care system for too long.

Another lesson emerges from the responses of all the community benefits programs to the effects of market competition and tight budgets. The extreme example of this, of course, was the experience at HPHC, but all the programs could look back wistfully to halcyon days of easier funding and less accountability. All the programs we studied had learned quickly how to look for alternative sources of funding. For example, many of Holy Cross's programs were initially internally supported with seed money, but, over time, many were able to receive larger and more sustainable funding from state and federal agencies. The internal commitment to community benefits as a matter of self-identity and corporate culture leads exemplary organizations to stick with projects whenever possible and work to find the resources to continue them, even through hard financial times.

Competitive and financial pressures also led every organization we spoke with to implement some plan to make their community benefits programs more coherent, organized, and accountable. Community benefit programs among these organizations must now be managed with the same diligent search for waste as that undertaken in every other department. In addition, financial pressures have catalyzed a shift from a relatively passive to a much more active process of prioritization within community benefit programs. Synergy, alignment, and coordination are now sought in every step the organization takes, and community benefits are no longer an exception. Group Health's restructuring, Holy Cross's financial accounting, and HPHC's refocusing of priorities all demonstrate that, among U.S. health-care organizations, the adolescence of community benefit programs is at an end; they have had to grow up quickly and now must be able to play at the same table as every other constituency in the organization.

A lingering question that our investigation was unable to address completely is whether for-profit health-care organizations can and should establish the same degree of community solidarity and empowerment in their community benefits programs. There are for-profit health plans that do provide community benefits, including free care and many of the specific types of programs we describe among nonprofit organizations. Nevertheless, for-profit corporations face certain intrinsic barriers. They tend not to be geographically localized in particular communities and are more likely to have diffuse networks spread out nationally or over large regions. They tend to grow, contract, buy, or be sold, more often than nonprofit companies. As a result, for-profit organizations often cannot identify easily with a particular community. In addition, without the background statutory requirements that oblige nonprofit organizations to contribute to the community welfare, for-profit corporations have a harder time justifying community benefit expenditures to shareholders. The need for marketing they may understand, but pure community benefit programs are a much tougher sell. Economic pressures on for-profit corporations certainly can be just as intense as they are for any other health-care organization, and the rationale that "we pay taxes, so the rest is expendable" may be irresistible. It may even be right. In competitive markets it seems too much to expect that for-profit companies, paying their fair share of taxes, should, in addition, contribute to community benefit programs in amounts comparable to that of nonprofits.

But although we do not cite any specific examples in our book, we believe that community solidarity and empowerment are not values that are by nature foreign to for-profit health-care companies. Nor do we believe that for-profit companies need to throw up their hands and capitulate to a minimalist approach to community benefit. To survive, the values of solidarity and empowerment will need persuasive voices to come to their defense when the values of stewardship and economic success are also on the table. The same is true within all organizations. A little leadership can go a long way. But the underlying lesson of this chapter is that health-care organizations of quite different stripes can create their own sense of community solidarity and empowerment in a variety of ways, in different health-care markets. They can make a significant difference in the lives of individuals and in the texture of our social commitments to each other in our communities. Organizations can achieve these ethical ends through good times and bad. We hope the examples in this chapter will give more organizations the confidence to try.

NOTES

1. *A.P. Smith Mfg. Co.* vs. *Barlow* 98 A2d 581, appeal dismissed 346 U.S. 861 (1953).
2. Delaware General Corporation Law §122.
3. California Corporations Code §207(e).

8

THE CONFIDENTIALITY OF PERSONAL
HEALTH INFORMATION

On August 2, 2000, a large nonprofit HMO, IntegraCare, accidentally sent responses to 858 customers' e-mails to the wrong members. The members whose confidentiality was breached were using IntegraCare's on-line service to make appointments and discuss sensitive health matters with doctors. The problem occurred as the HMO was upgrading software for its on-line system to handle increased traffic. IntegraCare characterized some of the information that was sent to the wrong members as "very sensitive" (Brubaker, 2000).

After suffering a work-related injury to her wrist, a California woman authorized IntegraCare to release information pertaining to her ailment to her employer. When she later had the opportunity to review her medical record, she found that the file sent to her employer contained her *entire* medical history, including records on recent fertility treatment and pregnancy loss that were completely unrelated to the wrist ailment (McCarthy, 1999).

IntegraCare is a fictitious name, but these cases are real and in the public domain. They highlight a growing concern about the confidentiality of personal medical information in an age of large health-care organizations and dizzying technological advances. Confidentiality, however, has always been central to medical ethics, extending back to the time of the Hippocratic oath. Confidentiality is a deeply held value in medicine and a pillar of the patient–doctor relationship. It is generally agreed that health care is improved when patients feel safe confiding sensitive medical information to their caregivers and that patients who fear their private stories will be disclosed may withhold pertinent information (Ethical Force Program, 2000). But how can patients be sure that the information they provide will remain confidential? In the past, they had only the personal integrity of their individual doctors to worry about. But now, personal information of all kinds is recorded electronically and seems to pass through semipermeable membranes to places and organizations of which we have little knowledge. Anyone who has received unwanted e-mail from a merchant who obtained the e-mail address from some unknown source has felt the uneasy feeling of being watched, and even invaded. As health information joins the cavalcade of available personal electronic data, many are asking, what are the legitimate uses of personal health information outside the immediate clinical setting? And, even when personal health information is shared with others for good reasons, how can the appropriate level of privacy for individuals be protected? The struggle to define boundaries between respect for individual privacy and the collection of health data for legitimate uses has led to widespread debate over how competing ethical values can be appropriately balanced.

The public is clearly worried about the status of this balancing act. A 1999 survey by the California Health Care Foundation found that one in five Americans believes his or her health information has been used or disclosed inappropriately, and one in six now engages in some form of privacy-protective behavior when they seek, receive, or pay for health care.[1] The likelihood that personal genetic information will someday soon be part of each patient's medical record has only heightened anxieties. At the same time, however, computerized medical information systems have been shown to have important public benefits, such as reducing mistakes, lowering costs, and improving the quality of care (Gostin, 1998; Monane et al., 1998). As a result of these positive features, there is increasing demand from outside the clinical setting—from insurers, public health agencies, oversight bodies, researchers, and employers—for access to patient information for a variety of purposes, including quality improvement, prevention, credentialing, marketing, and medical research.

Can ethical frameworks help organizations balance competing visions of the privacy and the usefulness of medical information? How can attention devoted to privacy issues enhance trust between health care organizations and their members? These issues are at the core of this chapter exploring health plans' alternative approaches to member confidentiality.

BACKGROUND

In recent years, there have been numerous efforts within both the public and private sectors to develop standards for health-care confidentiality. The results have been diverse and inconsistent, however, and there has been little guidance on how to implement proposed guidelines. Even after the passage of the federal Health Insurance Portability and Accountability Act (HIPAA) in 1996—the legislation that was supposed to establish comprehensive new privacy guidelines for all health care organizations—subsequent questions, alterations, and vague interpretations have left many elements unclear.

With limited exceptions, most health plans have restricted their efforts with regard to confidentiality to whatever is necessary to comply strictly with applicable regulations. Organizations that have embraced more comprehensive programs have done so voluntarily, placing confidentiality high on the list of organizational priorities. We contend that these organizations have reaped broad benefits from this emphasis, as outlined later in this chapter. Combined with a current shift toward increasing regulation, there are compelling reasons for health plans to consider embracing confidentiality as an important organizational value, instead of simply a compliance concern.

State-level privacy regulations have existed for some time. State laws developed in a piecemeal fashion and were enacted at different points in time to address a wide variety of scenarios and public health concerns (Pritts et al., 1999). Regulations tend to differ extensively across jurisdictions and vary according to the type, source, and holder of the data at issue. Among the more common rules are those addressing the right of access to information, conditions of disclosure, disease-specific requirements to protect particularly sensitive information, and the creation and use of government records. In most states, the result is a patchwork system of protections, with many gaps. It is interesting to note that, within state regulations, an ethical duty to maintain confidentiality is often presumed. Many statutes do not impose an affirmative duty of confidentiality upon clinicians or organizations, but do impose a penalty for breaches of confidentiality (Pritts et al., 1999).

At the federal level, enactment of comprehensive privacy protections has been a politically divisive struggle. As mentioned, HIPAA requires many health-care organizations to comply with new privacy guidelines by April 2003. The legislation originally intended Congress to promulgate specific regulations. After lengthy debate, however, Congress was unable to reach consensus, and the task fell to the Secretary of Health and Human Services. The final regulations apply to health plans, including HMOs, health insurers, and group health plans, as well as health-care "clearinghouses" and certain providers. However, they do not apply to many other entities that collect and maintain health information, such as employers, life insurers, researchers, and public health officials. In addition, the Bush Administration has been active in reinterpreting some of the key provisions of HIPAA. Thus, while HIPAA creates certain new rights (such as access to a patient's own medical records), critics contend that their scope is too narrow, their interpretation a moving target, and that, overall, they fail to constitute a comprehensive set of federal protections for medical information.

Despite this criticism, HIPAA regulations are the most affirmative privacy obligations to date placed on many health-care organizations. HIPAA is forcing many organizations to look closely at their confidentiality programs for the first time, creating an ideal opportunity to go beyond compliance and incorporate ethics into business strategy. Looking at best practices of organizations that have already followed this path can provide guidance to those whose work is at an earlier stage.

At the same time that HIPAA privacy rules were being debated in Congress, a variety of oversight agencies, trade organizations, and other entities in the private sector began promoting voluntary standards and model principles of confidentiality. Many of these efforts reflect, as one report noted, "fundamental concerns over how health care is adapting to the information revolution" (Ethical Force Program, 2000). The Model State Public Health Privacy Project, for example, has developed model health privacy legislation for states, and Georgetown University's Health Privacy Project in 1999 issued a report, *Best Principles for Health Privacy* (Health Privacy Project, 1999). As part of its Putting Patients First initiative, the American Association of Health Plans recently revised its recommended member policies on protecting patient privacy and record confidentiality. The National Committee for Quality Assurance has incorporated privacy standards in its accreditation reviews. And many other organizations, including the American Medical Association, American Bar Association, and National Association of Insurance Commissioners have similarly addressed or adopted health privacy recommendations (Ethical Force Program, 2000).

As organizations adjust to ever-changing technology and prepare to comply with both voluntary standards and with HIPAA, little is known about how some organizations have already developed particularly strong confidentiality policies or have created a *culture* of confidentiality. What values are considered? Which stakeholders have input? What are the benefits of going beyond a compliance model of confidentiality? Much can be learned by examining how certain health plans have navigated the landscape of technological innovation, medical advances, and regulatory standards that converge around this issue.

ETHICAL VALUES AND CENTRAL ETHICAL OBLIGATIONS

The term *confidentiality* can have a wide variety of meanings in different health plans. When we speak of medical privacy or confidentiality (and we use these terms interchangeably), we refer to the collection, use, and/or disclosure of personal health information by health-care organizations and their affiliated clinical practitioners. There may be legitimate reasons for personal health information to be released to those outside the immediate clinical setting (particularly in deidentified form), and we believe that an ethical approach to confidentiality does not evaluate organizations solely on the extent to which they prevent or allow this. Instead, as in our previous chapters, we focus our ethical analysis largely at policy-making processes, guided by several normative central ethical obligations. We look at the extent of an organization's conscious awareness of inherent tensions between ethical values in confidentiality, as well as its process of developing programs to address and manage these tensions.

Our list of central ethical obligations in the domain of confidentiality is shown in Table 8–1. Ultimately, we are interested in whether an organization uses a balanced approach to formulate confidentiality strategies. We do not contend that there is any single, correct approach to protect patient confidentiality while fostering positive health-care initiatives. Nor do we focus solely on a consumer-protection view of confidentiality. Rather, we believe that the *thoughtfulness and thoroughness* of an organization's approach—even if its ultimate program prioritizes one set of claims over others—may serve to demonstrate that its confidentiality program is inherently ethical.

We contend that there are legitimate ethical values that support the use of personal health information in initiatives to improve public health and reshape health care—such as community health information networks, outcomes analyses, disease management—and even unforeseen initiatives such as the fight against bioterrorism. In considerations of confidentiality policies, organizations in competitive markets will also value the economic importance of good relationships with purchasers, vendors, and consultants. These outside agents may have strong or weak claims to personal health information, and health care organizations will feel a legitimate business desire to give them the information they want, when they want it, and in the format they want it.

Table 8–1. Central ethical obligations for confidentiality

THE CONFIDENTIALITY POLICIES OF EXEMPLARY ETHICAL ORGANIZATIONS MUST:

1. Be created with input from multiple stakeholders (members, physicians, employers or other payers, researchers, and/or public health officials).
2. Be clearly communicated to stakeholders, including the rationale behind their creation.
3. Show an appreciation for different types of medical information, with different levels of sensitivity (e.g., mental health or sexually transmitted diseases).
4. Balance legitimate interests in obtaining information.
5. Prioritize the risk to individuals of leaking identifiable clinical information.
6. Include provisions for adequate training of personnel in confidentiality policies and procedures.
7. Have their impact measured, with some mechanism for ongoing reflection that includes input from stakeholders.
8. Incorporate flexibility or some mechanism for handling special cases.
9. Require that the organization only share personal health information with partners who commit explicitly to the same level of sensitivity regarding confidentiality.

In direct opposition to the values supporting legitimate and semilegitimate uses of personal health information is the value of confidentiality as a bedrock of protection of vulnerable persons. We posit that a patient's right to privacy is extremely important, particularly where sensitive issues such as mental health, communicable disease, or reproductive history are involved. Out of concern that disclosure of personal health information could result in embarrassment, stigmatization, or discrimination, we contend that the uses of personal health information should be designed to extract only the most narrow set of information needed, process that information in deidentified formats whenever possible, and adequately safeguard the information from additional or accidental exposure to others.

Different stakeholders in the health-care system embrace critical values and interests around medical data that often conflict yet must be prioritized and balanced in some fashion. As we learn about various organizations' approaches to confidentiality, we have sought to understand how well the structures and processes they adopt achieve the central ethical obligations we have outlined above. Implementing an exemplary confidentiality policy requires an organization to go beyond strict compliance with relevant laws and guidelines, actively promoting a culture of trust and confidentiality through all levels of the company. Clearly defined and legitimate confidentiality policies are essential for sustaining the trust of patients and the public. Organizations that have devoted considerable effort to developing and instilling privacy protections have much to offer others who are still struggling to understand the key choices and best options in this domain.

EXEMPLARY PRACTICES

In each of the examples described below of exemplary organizational approaches to confidentiality, the tension between ethical values was made explicit, and multiple stakeholders were invited into the process of deliberation. Then, when priorities had been established and practical solutions for ethical tensions fully developed, the ultimate set of confidentiality policies was integrated into the business strategy of the organization. It is important to note, however, that each of the organizations described below came to embrace confidentiality issues for very different reasons. What they share that is exemplary is an approach to resolving confidentiality tensions that is comprehensive, practical, and fluid.

The Harvard Pilgrim Health Care Model: A Catalyzing Crisis Leads to New Protections for the Medical Record

Much of the excellence in Harvard Pilgrim Health Care's (HPHC's) confidentiality policies came after an explosive incident in 1995 involving the health plan's staff-model HMO. A brief review of this background sets the stage for the organization's current approach to confidentiality.

HPHC had a long tradition of providing integrated health-care services. Part of the organization's vision included an electronic medical record that would allow seamless care wherever a patient was seen within the system—any clinician would have access to all clinical encounters, test results, prescriptions, allergies, etc. The electronic medical record was viewed as central to how the organization cared for its patients and a critical feature of its business model. HPHC's commitment to integrated care included mental health, and thus, mental health information was also part of the electronic medical record. Mental health clinicians did not put extensive notes in the record, but often did indicate personal information, as well as diagnoses they felt pertinent for other clinicians to know about.

It was against this backdrop that, in 1995, an article appeared in the *Boston Globe* detailing the complaint of an HPHC patient, whose mental health background, told to a psychiatrist under the assumption that it was confidential, was repeated to her by an obstetrician who had read it in her electronic medical record. The article sparked great concern among HPHC patients, as well as a flurry of negative attention to the health plan and its prized medical record system.

The health plan's immediate response was to announce that it would completely segregate mental health information from the rest of the clinical record. However, HPHC clinicians quickly complained that this action left them blind to important clinical information and would be detrimental to care. HPHC was thus catalyzed by two critical stakeholders—its members and its clinicians—into a longer, more reflective process of examining both the structure and use of its electronic medical record system. This process resulted in a rigorous, ongoing effort to find ways to balance conflicting needs and values regarding access to sensitive clinical information.

To launch the process, a broad-based HPHC confidentiality committee, composed of clinicians, computer experts, health plan staff, and community members, convened focus groups of members and providers to deliberate about meaningful distinctions between different types of personal health information and various steps that could be taken to safeguard confidentiality. Over time, important compromises were reached by meeting the concerns of each group. For example, psychiatric medications were ultimately reinstated in the medical record; depression diagnoses also were made visible in the record to all clinicians; and psychiatric hospitalizations and visits were once again listed. New computer systems were created to allow clinicians with mental health user codes to gain access to more detailed mental health information. Medical record audit trails were also created to allow the review of all individuals who had accessed the medical record. The breakthrough concept embraced by all participants in the deliberation process was a search for degrees of freedom instead of an all-or-nothing approach to personal health information in the medical record. Thus, personal health information was divided into different types according to the degree of risk to the patient of their disclosure. Working with these categories, the group was able to define zones of safety that would be accorded each type of medical information. This conceptualization represented a way to find legitimate compromises between the group's competing values and perspectives on confidentiality.

Today, confidentiality policies at the clinical practice level have reached an apex at the former HPHC staff-model practice, now known as Harvard Vanguard Medical Associates (HVMA). Largely as a result of all the work triggered by the 1995 *Boston Globe* article, HVMA confidentiality policies and programs have been prominent and remain firmly entrenched within the practice. HVMA policy explicitly recognizes key ethical tensions up front, stating,

> We recognize that there will be situations in which the patient's need for privacy will conflict with the clinician's "need to know." In those situations we seek to balance the conflicting needs protecting the patient's right to privacy without compromising our ability to provide safe and effective medical care.

Among the features of HVMA's strategy for achieving this goal are:

- Documentation guidelines for physicians, with each new physician employee required to undergo confidentiality training and pass a written test as part of orientation.
- Employee-wide training, including the requirement to view a video on confidentiality at orientation.
- Specific guidelines regarding appointments (e.g., "The patient's presence in a Health Center is itself a piece of confidential information").
- Consideration of disposal methods for medical records.
- Specific computerized methods to safeguard confidentiality, including audit trails so that members can tell who has been reading their charts.
- Direct consideration of issues pertaining to minors.
- Special categorization of clinical material that is particularly sensitive (e.g., HIV testing, abortions). Information in these categories is not released unless specifically authorized by the patient.
- Provisions that dictations that contain especially sensitive matter must be listed under a diagnostic code that is screened out under the provisions above (so that, for example, HIV-positive status cannot be mentioned under the diagnostic code for sore throat).
- Safeguards ensuring that mental health codes and dictations are not visible to non-mental-health clinicians.
- Systematic confidentiality audit processes conducted in the clinical units.
- Communuication of confidentiality policies to patients.

When HVMA was split off from HPHC, leaving HPHC as an insurer without a direct provider component, it might have seemed natural that HPHC's concern with and attention to confidentiality would wane. This is far from the case. As a health plan, HPHC maintains a high-profile and comprehensive confidentiality policy that targets all staff, stating in its preamble,

> Safeguarding patients' medical information, our staff's employment information, and information with respect to proprietary business matters is not only a legal require- ment, but also an important ethical obligation. . . . All HPHC staff have a responsi- bility to recognize the special relationship of trust between us and our patients and must safeguard all medical information and/or personal information about patients.

The policy clearly defines which medical information is considered sensitive and, notably, recognizes the unique status of individuals who are both HPHC patients *and* employees.

These policies at HVMA and HPHC go far beyond a compliance approach to confidentiality. We believe that there are three key themes in the combined work over the years by HVMA-HPHC that have particular merit from an ethical stand- point, as well as significant business benefits. First, the *Boston Globe* incident triggered a keen *awareness of ethical tensions in confidentiality* that has been retained by both organizations. HPHC embraced a bilateral commitment to pa- tient concerns *and* to clinician requests for access to data critical for patient care. This approach represented a departure from a strict "consumer protection" view of confidentiality and preserved HPHC's laudable commitment to an integrated, accessible record of medical care.

Second, HPHC included *multiple perspectives* in considering the issues and creating its policies. The dialogue between diverse stakeholders was felt to have a clarifying effect and to have provided new opportunities for effective compro- mise, as well as entirely new systems for safeguarding patient confidentiality and the quality of care.

Finally, the organization *openly deliberated* the issues involved in structuring a privacy program. These last two pieces of HPHC's approach had value for the organization, even apart from the resulting confidentiality policies. The inclusive, democratic methods employed served as early and successful lessons in what would become the central features of HPHC's organizational ethics program.

Today HPHC is struggling, as are other organizations, with the issue of how to implement its confidentiality policies across an increasingly diffuse physician network. There have also been some signs of attention fatigue. For example, rou- tine confidentiality audits within clinical areas have now ceased. Despite these challenges, however, both HVMA and HPHC retain a keen appreciation for the importance of confidentiality to patient trust, and continuing discussions about the evolution of policies and systems regarding confidentiality are frequently heard within both organizations.

One of the notable lessons from the HPHC story concerns the genesis of the organization's efforts to address privacy issues. The extensive policies developed by the former staff-model group originated in response to unfavorable publicity regarding the health plan's state-of-the-art electronic medical record. While the confidentiality program began as a grassroots response to this incident, first addressing only information contained within the medical record, it evolved into a thorough, far-reaching set of principles and procedures that affect not just clinicians but the entire organization. From HPHC we know that it may be risky for an organization to ignore privacy issues until forced to examine them. Many healthcare organizations are just beginning to consider carefully their confidentiality strategies and are relying on compliance with HIPAA, National Committee for Quality Assurance (NCQA), and other legal or accreditation parameters as sufficient involvement in the issue. But a strong confidentiality program, developed with input from and embraced by multiple stakeholders, can be a cornerstone of developing trust both within and outside an organization.

Confidentiality as an Organizational Priority

In contrast with HPHC, Group Health Cooperative of Puget Sound had no public crisis that pushed it to focus on confidentiality. Instead, Group Health made an affirmative decision in 1998 to readdress its confidentiality policies as a result of the increasing computerization of its medical record system, as well as the length of time that had passed since the health plan had last evaluated the issue.

As an initial step in assessing its existing policies, Group Health reconstituted and broadened its confidentiality and security council (CSC), a body that includes representatives from the medical staff, the behavioral health, information technology, and human resources departments, and the health plan's membership. Group Health's goal was to ensure that this group included a broad mix of backgrounds and perspectives. When certain issues were reviewed, such as those regarding research and mental health, adjunct members were invited to join the CSC to contribute their special interest and/or expertise in the area.

As the CSC evaluated how to approach confidentiality issues, it established one overriding principle as the basis for all of Group Health's policies on confidentiality: the concept of legitimate "business need to know." This principle emerged out of CSC's reading of the literature on privacy, but held particular appeal because it could be applied across the entire organization, including physicians' offices. The CSC determined that, while specific guidelines would be devised to fit certain situations, this principle would be the foundation for all future considerations of the confidentiality of patient information.

As envisioned by Group Health, "business need to know" asks each individual employee to exercise his or her best judgment to determine whether access to or use of patient information can be directly justified by a legitimate business need.

In addition to having an extensive list of specific situations in which certain information can be used, "business need to know" seeks to instill in all employees an active questioning process that can be more responsive to the nuances of particular situations. As a guiding principle, "business need to know" is meant to stir employees at all levels to a new awareness of the ethical tensions in viewing and disseminating member information, reaching above and beyond the limited power of written rules and guidelines.

Group Health reinforces its commitment to confidentiality through multiple avenues. The "business need to know" concept is introduced to all new employees through a confidentiality statement signed at the time of hire, as well as a video shown to all new employees. There is an on-line training program for hospitals, and clinics can request on-site confidentiality/security training. All computer classes include a brief introduction on the importance of confidentiality and security, often with a video. The Group Health staff newsletter reinforces the concept on a regular basis. New doctors receive extensive training on the issue. Group Health's policies have also been posted on its intranet, distributed by e-mail, and sent out in directed messages to all clinicians.

In addition to stressing the concept of "business need to know" through the measures above, Group Health has developed specific interventions aimed at confidentiality:

- Specific policies guide the sharing of information related to minors.
- There is a policy regarding the disposal of records and confidential documents.
- A separate program identifies and disposes of confidential waste—differentiating between confidential paper waste (which is shredded/recycled), confidential "other" (e.g., pill bottles), and regular garbage.
- Limited audit trails exist within the clinical information system.
- Regular communications inform members of policies regarding the collection, use, and protection of information.
- Special identification and protections exist for mental-health and HIV/AIDS information.

Group Health's strategy also incorporates a specific approach to handling requests for data that will be sent to outside parties such as vendors and purchasers. Most requests must be routed through the CSC, and the information security department performs a security analysis. There is also a process for handling access requests by nonclinical staff, such as billing personnel. Through these mechanisms, Group Health seeks to establish a uniform process for ensuring that patient information leaving the organization cannot be used for purposes it believes would threaten patient confidentiality.

One of the most distinctive features of Group Health's confidentiality program is a detailed access matrix that delineates which staff may access specific pieces of the organization's information databases. The matrix divides staff—including administrative, professional, and clinical personnel—into multiple categories, each with approval for access to specific types of protected information. The access matrix reflects policy, but also describes actual structural barriers that were designed through user IDs and other computer firewall systems to limit individual access to specific types of information. As such, it is the most concrete—yet evolving—manifestation of Group Health's consensus on "business need to know."

It is notable that, from the outset, Group Health asked itself how it could do better than mere compliance with NCQA guidelines in addressing confidentiality. The organization believes that NCQA regulations deal with the nuts and bolts of privacy protections and not the overall conceptualization of confidentiality. In contrast, we found that concern for confidentiality permeates the culture of Group Health's organization at all levels and is particularly noteworthy with regard to its inclusion of physicians. The idea that physicians should be part of a universal confidentiality strategy flows naturally from Group Health's history and culture of close partnership with its providers.

Group Health's approach to confidentiality embraces many of the values we contend are important for ethical practice in this area. First, the concept of "business need to know" evolved from an interactive group of multiple stakeholders with diverse perspectives. This process yielded policies that are both sensitive to and more likely to be embraced by the variety of individuals impacted. Moreover, it preserves the cultures of cooperation and trust on which the organization rests. Second, Group Health repeatedly and extensively communicates its policies to stakeholders through a variety of mechanisms. Policies are thus accessible to interested parties, and the organization demonstrates its accountability in this domain. Third, Group Health has been active in measuring the effectiveness of its confidentiality training through the use of evaluation forms.

There are two particularly important features of Group Health's confidentiality strategy from which other organizations might benefit. The first is the consistency with which it has developed the concept of "business need to know" as a method for instilling a *culture of reflection and awareness* when it comes to questions surrounding the use and sharing of patient information. "Business need to know" shines as a useful approach that goes far beyond the development of a rote script of confidentiality scenarios and policies. Individuals acting within this parameter could be expected to exercise laudable initiative in managing unusual and novel circumstances in an ethical manner. We do recognize that in actual practice, of course, "business need to know" could degenerate into a relativistic and even self-interested approach, one in which each individual could selectively tailor his or her definition of "need to know" according to the situation.

The second specific element of Group Health's program worthy of emulation is the *access matrix*. Both conceptually and in practice, this is an excellent way of making visible the protections and contingencies that Group Health has built into its computer systems to safeguard patient information. As a tool for cross-organizational discussion, and as a method for making eminently clear what the safeguards are, the access matrix could be successively adopted at all kinds of health-care organizations. Consumers and interest groups wanting to understand the status of organizational confidentiality protections could be easily introduced to any system through this single kind of document.

There remain a number of significant issues and challenges to Group Health's approach. These include enforcing uniform sanctions for violations and ensuring that policies are incorporated into the network and business partner contracts to create a chain of trust. Despite the tremendous integration of its efforts across clinical and administrative lines in the organization, Group Health's greatest challenge in confidentiality remains its clinicians. Many clinicians seem to believe that any time they want to see a patient's information—for any reason—they have a legitimate "business need to know." Coalescing the worldview of clinicians with administrative policies is a challenge for all health-care organizations, and Group Health is aware it will need to keep working in this area.

LESSONS LEARNED

There are key underlying differences between the approaches to confidentiality embraced by HPHC and Group Health. At the outset, the impetus for each organization's efforts strongly influenced its final structure. At HPHC, the organization reacted to an external event with a grassroots effort to balance each stakeholder's values and needs. As policies were developed, they filtered upward through the organization, were embraced by the leadership, and became embedded in the organization's culture as it evolved into new corporate entities. With Group Health, a top-down initiative began with a formal review of existing policies and resulted in a comprehensive set of programs and documents that filtered outward through the organization's many branches.

Despite these differences, there are two important principles underlying both organizations' confidentiality programs that offer lessons for organizations new to privacy issues. First, each approach incorporated a *conscious recognition* of the tensions involved in developing a confidentiality strategy—competing claims were explicitly stated and became the cornerstone of each organization's program. Neither organization chose to take an all-or-nothing approach, which could have emphasized either a patient-protection focus or domination of the health plan's need for access to data. Second, each organization developed an extremely thorough program addressing privacy issues. Each went significantly beyond regulatory obligations in developing its safeguards, actively embracing and promoting confidentiality as a key corporate value.

Both of these features can be embraced by a wide variety of health-care entities in developing confidentiality programs. The culture of trust and respect that results from the process of defining and considering values before drafting specific policies can only serve to benefit any organization—for-profit or nonprofit, large or small—that is in the business of promoting health.

As health-care organizations strive over coming years to comply with new federal health privacy regulations, they have an opportunity to add significant value to the task. Both HPHC and Group Health view their confidentiality policies as a vehicle for enhancing member and practitioner trust—a goal that a compliance-oriented approach to meeting HIPAA requirements will surely fail to achieve. Neither HPHC nor Group Health found the design of a substantial privacy program to be sufficient; each put substantial energy into *implementation* as well. While we recognize that market pressures will tempt many organizations to narrow the scope of their HIPAA programs to strict regulatory compliance, we suggest that this approach is shortsighted. The range of health conditions requiring special confidentiality concerns is likely to expand—genetic information and mental-health data are just two rapidly growing areas. Similarly, the technology of personal health information will certainly continue to evolve rapidly, presenting ever more challenges—and opportunities—for controlling the use of that information. From the Hippocratic Oath to HIPAA, confidentiality as a core ethical concern in health care has been with us and is likely to remain. Embracing confidentiality as an organizational priority and an opportunity for inclusive deliberation is a positive step for all health-care organizations to consider.

NOTE

1. Such behavior may include paying out of pocket for care, intentionally seeing multiple providers to avoid the creation of a consolidated record, giving inaccurate or incomplete information on a medical history, asking a doctor not to write down the health problem or record a less serious or embarrassing condition, and even not seeking care to avoid disclosure to an employer. (California HealthCare Foundation, survey conducted by Princeton Survey Research Associates, January 1999.)

9

THE PERENNIAL ETHICAL
CHALLENGES OF HEALTH CARE
IN COMPETITIVE SYSTEMS

> Visionary companies . . . don't see it as a choice between living to
> their values or being pragmatic; they see it as a challenge to find
> pragmatic solutions and behave consistent with their core values.
> James Collins and Jerry Porras*

In this chapter we return to the central reality guiding this book: as important as health is, it is not the only socially valued goal, nor are technical health-care services the only means of improving health. Thus, every advanced health-care system must cope with the ethical tensions generated by considering costs as well as the quality of health care. Priorities must be set. Difficult choices have to be made, often producing tense compromise or open disappointment. Into this atmosphere may enter a toxic combination of suspicion and resentment when individual and organizational profits are made part of the delicate balancing act. The result is a powerful ethical and political challenge: how can patients, providers, and the public trust the legitimacy and fairness of the organizations that provide health care in competitive systems? This has been the focus of our work.

Every advanced health-care system has wrestled with this problem. Sweden and the other Nordic countries, along with the Netherlands, have convened national groups to delineate explicit ethical criteria for how to distribute health care fairly. Great Britain and Canada, on the other hand, have had some level of public discussion about the problem of scarcity and limits to care, but have relied instead on their well-entrenched combination of universal insurance and implicit forms of limit setting (Daniels and Sabin, 2002). But even with national commissions

*Collins, J. C. and Porras, J. I. (1994). *Built to Last*. New York: Harper-Collins Publishers, p. 62.

and universal insurance, setting health-care priorities and rationing remains an unavoidably messy, conflict-ridden, ultimately tragic social process. Even countries with deep roots of solidarity and public deliberation face the perennial challenge of establishing legitimacy for the difficult decisions that must be made in health care.

The United States, of course, has taken another path into the same wilderness. After the very visible failure of the Clinton reform effort in the early 1990s, the American public was left somewhat dazed and confused, bombarded with sound bites, but bereft of an understanding of the reality of health care limits. Large private and governmental purchasers of health-care services lost what little hope they may have had that political leadership would soon break the logjam. But they also knew that costs were rising fast, at a pace that could not long be sustained. Purchasers needed an answer at hand and turned to the only mechanism to control costs that seemed feasible in the near term: the market. Managed care was to have its day in the sun.

Managed care, of course, has meant many things to different people over time. But over the past decade, through the smoke and fire of constant mergers and acquisitions, public distrust, and clinician disdain, we can see in the experience of managed care in the United States the traces, and, one hopes, the lessons, of a social experiment. During this experiment, health care would be shaped without explicit priorities or deliberative process. Private health-care organizations, many of them constituted along for-profit lines, and all competing in fierce, winner-take-all environments, would bear an increasing responsibility for reining in escalating costs while maintaining or even improving the delivery of care. They would have the power of the purse and the mandate to use it. But patients, physicians, and the public, although cardholders at this high-stakes table, were not to understand the true nature of the game. The charade that health resources were unlimited would continue. For who would sign on with the first health-care organization acknowledging limits and promising to ration care wisely? Based on an implicit faith in the ability of markets to maximize value, insurance companies were ceded the power to set priorities and define the limits of health care. But they were to wield their power without true public sanction or understanding.

The subsequent events that have dominated the experiment with managed care in the United States are well known. The reorganization and recontracting of the American health-care system meant that there was a lot of money to be made in the short term, a realization that did not often encourage examples of the highest form of human or organizational conduct. In Boston, for example, a widely distributed analysis by a respected consulting organization heralded the existence of a "3 Billion Dollar Catch." Apparently there was an "extra" $3 billion each year being spent on health care in the Boston marketplace that was not going to last long. Someone was going to get it. Would it be the purchasers? Or perhaps the HMOs? Even the hospitals had a shot at keeping it. It was a race with a big pot of gold at the finish line. And reading the analysis, one couldn't help agreeing with the author that the race would go to the swiftest, most aggressive, toughest player in the field. Across the United States, the race for the money became the most important health-care issue. Concerns about access to care for millions of uninsured slipped off the radar screen, and even the original vision of managed care, that of population-based systems to foster higher quality of care, could not hope to hold a candle to the drama and the intensity of the day-to-day struggle for "covered lives," market share dominance, and enormous profit.

Thus, across much of the United States, the story of managed care can be told as a series of stories of villains and victims, high finance and low behavior. However, the U.S. experience can also be told as a story about facing problems and searching for solutions. Not unlike the Provincial Health Plans in the Canadian single-payer system and the District Health Authorities in the U.K. National Health Service, every health-care organization in the United States during the heyday of managed care has faced the dilemma of how to provide the best health care possible within resource constraints. Capitation and other forms of risk sharing have meant that not only insurers but provider organizations have often had to face this ongoing tension. In the diverse health care markets across the country, each with its own unique set of competitors, historical patterns, and current realities, we can examine the results from many different "laboratories" in which health care organizations sought pragmatic responses to this challenge. What can we learn from the experience of organizations during this tumultuous time? No single health-care organization is perfect; many, however, can claim a few policies, structures, or processes, often created anew after the cleansing fire of a previous public disaster, that embody exemplary ethical features. This book is based on the premise that these exemplary practices come with lessons learned and insights acquired that can move us forward in the perennial quest for legitimacy and ethical excellence in the face of health-care limits. What, then, have we learned?

THE ETHICAL QUALITY OF HEALTH-CARE
ORGANIZATIONS IN COMPETITIVE SYSTEMS

In this book we have presented examples and analyses of specific exemplary practices. What can these tell us more broadly about how to evaluate and promote the ethical quality of health-care organizations in competitive systems? All health-care organizations with limited resources face ethical challenges, but organizations trying to set priorities and balance ethical goods while competing in market systems carry a special burden. One way to conceptualize the ethical quality of health-care organizations under these circumstances is to separate the determinants of organizational ethical quality into four distinct elements (see Table 9–1). Some of these elements will be found to be relevant for health-care organizations

Table 9–1. The dimensions of ethical quality of health-care organizations facing constrained resources in a competitive system

DIMENSION OF ORGANIZATIONAL ETHICAL QUALITY	RELEVANT BEST PROJECT ETHICAL DOMAIN
Systems that foster exemplary achievement of primary ethical principles and tenets of medicine, e.g. autonomy, beneficence, nonmaleficence, and confidentiality.	Confidentiality
Systems to promote compliance with regulations, broader conceptions of organizational integrity, and an organizational capacity for reflection that allows appreciation of the ethical dimensions to operational strategy and decisions.	Organizational Ethics
Exemplary management of the ethical tension between the need for sustainable profit margins in a competitive market and the costs associated with:	
a. the traditional value of caring for the sickest, neediest patients. b. clinical autonomy (letting patients and doctors decide what resources to use and how). c. making contributions to an improved community.	a. Care of Vulnerable Populations b. Medical Necessity Determination c. Community Benefit
Exemplary achievement of collaborative decision-making relationships with physicians and patients. The elements of a collaborative patient–clinician relationship shared by organizations include:	Consumer Empowerment
a. honesty. b. respect for the values of others. c. provision of the information necessary for shared decision making. d. creation of systems for shared decision making. e. commitment to continuity of relationships.	

in any environment, while others will apply only to those at least partly exposed to a competitive and pluralistic system such as that found currently in the United States.

Most fundamentally, all health-care organizations are ethically accountable for their development or use of systems that affect the achievement of the primary goals and principles of medicine, i.e. beneficence, nonmaleficence, patient autonomy, and justice. Relevant to this dimension of ethical quality would be many of the health-care improvement initiatives that are the hallmark of most managed care organizations in the United States. For example, an HMO that develops a system of patient reminders to increase mammography, with the aim of preventing breast cancer deaths, can be said to show strength in this particular dimension of ethical quality. The same could be said for a hospital that creates a special program to reduce medical errors or a provider group that develops a program to foster patient-centered decision making in areas such as the management of early-stage prostate cancer or end-of-life care. Sometimes these clinical initiatives are ignored by ethicists who may consider them as belonging to the operational, and not the ethical, dimension of health-care organizations. But organizational attention is itself a limited resource, and when it is selectively and effectively turned toward the achievement of life-enhancing outcomes for patients, an organization is clearly exercising an ethical dimension of its functions.

From the group of ethical domains identified in the BEST project, confidentiality stands out as the one that links most naturally to this particular dimension of organizational ethical quality. A key attribute of the organizations in which we found models for exemplary practice in confidentiality was their conscious recognition that confidentiality was a central organizational concern. Confidentiality wasn't something that only doctors and nurses had to think about; it was part of a health-care organization's duty to its members and patients. As a result, significant organizational resources were dedicated to addressing stakeholder perspectives and to creating systems to manage the needs for clinical information in an ethically justifiable manner. In this regard, our findings and analysis of confidentiality programs provide a broadly applicable model: take the issue as a serious organizational concern; talk to and engage stakeholders within and outside the organization; reflect on the potential ethical dimensions of various alternatives; implement new approaches with humility and with an explicit mechanism for following the results and reflecting further on possible improvements. When organizations adopt this approach, be it toward confidentiality, end-of-life care programs, initiatives to reduce medical error, or any effort to improve patient care, they will likely create exemplary practices that enhance patient outcomes and trust.

A second dimension of organizational ethical quality that is common to health-care organizations in any environment is the dimension of organizational ethics itself. With the guidance of medical leaders, the BEST project identified organizational ethics as a specific ethical domain. During our investigation, we found great variation in the degree to which health-care organizations had developed effective internal systems to foster compliance with regulations and build throughout the organization a broader sense of integrity and an organizational capacity for reflection that allowed appreciation of the ethical dimensions of operational strategy and decisions. But, as the diverse exemplary practices we analyzed in Chapter 3 made clear, there is no one preordained road map through which an organization creates an effective infrastructure for organizational ethics. Diversity in organizational ethics is not to be regretted; it will be necessary in any pluralistic system of organizations with different histories, cultures, and missions. Organizational cultures can vary dramatically from faith-based, provider-dominated hospital systems to lean, for-profit insurers, and yet our investigation showed that all of these organizations can develop deep and effective structures for organizational ethics.

As we described in Chapter 3, we use the term *organizational ethics* to refer to the organization's efforts to *define* its own core values and mission, *identify* areas in which important values come into conflict, *seek* the best possible resolution of these conflicts, and *manage* its own performance to ensure that it acts in accord with espoused values. This is a definition that requires an organizational culture and volition that can sustain the focus to carry out these tasks. But it remains a predominantly procedural definition, one that, consistent with our pragmatic approach, would allow for diversity in the normative content of organizational ethics. Not every health-care organization must set the same relative priority on serving the indigent, nor does every organization need to find the exact same balance between short-term profit and long-term commitments to improving health.

If this is true, however, what remains, if anything, of normative standards and aspirations for organizational ethics? Our field work during the BEST project has reinforced our conviction that ethically admirable organizations must have a deeply held set of values that reasonable people would accept as appropriate to the active promotion of health and care of the sick. We will have more to say later in this chapter about our vision of the genesis and application of those values. For now, however, in considering organizational ethics, we stress the great importance of having procedural and structural components that can enable an organization to reflect, to appreciate the ethical components of operational strategy and decisions, and to act in consonance with its values.

Our experience working with many health-care organizations suggests that there is also a strong corollary between the ability of an organization, as an *organization*, to achieve this goal and its ability to foster the identical instincts and skills in *individuals* throughout the organization. Let us read our definition of organizational ethics again, thinking this time of what it would mean for an organization to have the ability to foster in *individuals* the skill to "define [their] own core values and mission, identify areas in which important values come into conflict, seek the best possible resolution of these conflicts, and manage [their] own performance to ensure that [they] act in accord with espoused values." Any organization would be proud to say that it takes a leading role in nurturing the formation of this skill in its employees. And for large health-care organizations, in which ethical values, in many guises, come into conflict in disparate parts of the company, it is essential that individuals have an independent capacity to see ethical conflict and manage it well. In some sense, this is where organizational ethics verges on the territory traditionally occupied by the concept of compliance, but, in fact, it is much more. Compliance magnified in the individual is integrity, a deep, although not blind, allegiance of the individual to the espoused dominant values of the organization and community. The ethically admirable health-care organization, therefore, must not only have defined ethics structures such as ethics committees and visible mission statements, it must also be governed and densely populated by persons of individual integrity.

Of virtues such as integrity much has been written. Corporate America has recently shown again that such basic virtues as honesty and integrity can become the victims of turbulent and competitive markets. Our analysis of health-care organizations leads us to believe that there is a symbiotic relationship between the formal structures of organizational ethics and the character virtues of individuals that often determines whether right or wrong is done. Formal opportunities to reflect on current dilemmas in light of past experience, the chance to hear the heartfelt convictions of stakeholders both inside and outside of the organization, explicit linkages between business decisions and specific organizational values— these experiences allow for the repetition and reinforcement of positive individual virtues. And, in a reciprocal fashion, positive individual virtues flow back to the organization as seminal events, war stories, and corporate legends that nourish an organizational culture of integrity. Health-care organizations in all environments, but especially those managing limited resources in competitive markets, can create an atmosphere of ethical excellence only by forging this kind of unbreakable alloy between the organization's ethical structures and the characters of its employees.

If the second dimension of organizational ethical quality is dominated by concerns for procedure, structure, and integrity, the third dimension contains greater normative weight. This dimension encompasses the family of focused ethical tensions faced by organizations that must balance care and costs in competitive markets, and often in national systems of care. Throughout the ethical domains and examples discussed in this book, an underlying ethical tension arises when organizations' values of care come into conflict with the need for sustainable profit margins. Simply put, care costs money, and organizations need profits to survive: "No margin, no mission."

Three of the ethical domains identified for the BEST project are direct examples of this tension: community benefit, care of vulnerable populations, and medical necessity determination. The domain of community benefit raises the question of how health-care organizations should view the balance between profits and their role as good corporate citizens. No matter whether an organization is structured as a for-profit or nonprofit corporation, the question remains, for the quantity and type of community benefit can range tremendously among comparable organizations.

Similarly, the ethical challenge of caring for vulnerable populations pits operating margins against the intrinsically higher costs of caring for the sickest, neediest patients. The economic model of prepaid care, which, at the organizational level, can support innovative systems for prevention, disease management, and patient-friendly alternatives to hospitalization, can equally encourage organizations to construct elaborate barriers to entry for sicker patients and to try to skim the healthiest part of the population off the top, leaving those with greater health risks to be cared for by others.

And, as we saw in Chapter 5, great ethical challenges arise in the conflict over medical necessity and other organizational approaches to medical policy. Managed care, by design, set out to rein in clinical autonomy—the freedom of clinicians and patients to use whatever medical resources they considered useful. During the halcyon days of managed care in the United States, many organizations felt that costs could be controlled largely through the rigorous application of evidence-based tools to weed out unnecessary and even dangerous medical care. This is a good, even noble, ideal. But the darker side of this vision is always with us in a competitive market system, certainly in the mind of the public. *Evidence-based*, at the population level, translates into *rationing* at the individual level. When the public is not an active partner in grappling with health-care limits, and when the profit of large, impersonal organizations is in the balance opposite sick patients' perceived health needs, the public will continue to doubt the ethical legitimacy of medical necessity determinations made by those organizations.

The ethical domains of care of vulnerable populations, community benefit, and medical necessity determination each provide core examples of the tension between important health care values and the drive of organizations to survive and grow. In the chapters dedicated to these domains, we have held to our pragmatic approach in presenting multiple paths toward ethically justifiable goals. But we have not forsaken normative content for the sake of an expedient survey of what seems to work in the marketplace. In the central ethical obligations of each chapter, we have provided important normative landmarks for organizations seeking ethical excellence. Among these normative ethical obligations we have included explicit statements of values that should be given priority by health-care organizations. Such values include communal solidarity, the identification of the care of vulnerable populations as part of the mission of the organization, and the value of supporting treating physicians in their role as advocates for their patients in benefit adjudication.

But even in these more focused ethical domains, the normative content of our analysis of specific values and their relative priority has remained relatively thin.

Instead, our normative contribution in these chapters arises largely in our consideration of the elements necessary for robust forms of procedural justice within organizations burdened with the setting of health-care limits. Community benefit, care of vulnerable populations, and medical necessity determination all arise as domains of ethical tension because of the underlying absence of agreement on broad principles of distributive justice that should govern the setting of priorities in a resource-limited, competitive system (Daniels and Sabin, 2002). There are universally acknowledged values of care, compassion, and focus on the individual sick person. There are other values of efficiency, population health, and wise stewardship of resources. Throwing in values of shareholder return and fidelity to employees adds even more layers of valid considerations. Were there societal consensus on fine-grained principles of justice that could be applied to determine the appropriate balance of these values in specific cases, there might be little moral controversy in health-care systems. But, lacking such principled consensus, modern societies and organizations must rely largely on procedural justice.

Working with Norman Daniels, James E. Sabin, an author of the present volume, has written previously to describe a framework for procedural justice that can provide the elusive legitimacy necessary for setting limits in health care (Daniels and Sabin, 1997; Sabin and Daniels, 1998; Daniels and Sabin, 2002). This framework is known as *accountability for reasonableness*. Because so many of the ethical challenges in organizational health care arise from the central problem of setting limits, the idea of accountability for reasonableness has contributed deeply to the specific central ethical obligations we have presented in each chapter of this book. According to this concept, four conditions are necessary for a decision-making process to meet the standards of legitimate procedural justice: publicity, relevance, revisability, and enforcement. First, rationales for key decisions must be made public. Not only must the decisions themselves be public, but the grounds for making them must be public as well. Publicity ensures transparency, a cornerstone of legitimacy, and is necessary for any kind of useful, shared learning over time by decision makers and the public. For example, as we pointed out in our chapter on medical necessity determination, innovative ways to use the Internet and other media to make the rationale for medical necessity decisions available to patients and physicians can contribute to exemplary achievement of the central ethical obligation to make this information public. Similarly, an organization's decision to limit its exposure to the care of vulnerable populations, or to direct its community benefit to one priority over another, should be accompanied with public disclosure of the reasons for such decisions.

The second condition of accountability for reasonableness requires that the rationales presented to justify key decisions must turn on evidence, reasons, and principles that fair-minded people can see are relevant to meeting health needs fairly under resource constraints. In other words, decisions in which there are competing ethical values must be justified by appeals to evidence, reasons, and principles that are accepted by fair-minded stakeholders as reasonable to consider in addressing the problem. For example, in medical necessity decisions it is easy to see that safety and efficacy would be viewed by all stakeholders as relevant. But what about cost and cost-effectiveness? At a minimum, certain ramifications of the methods used in cost-effectiveness analyses need to be explicitly addressed and agreed upon before cost-effectiveness can meet the standard of relevancy. What about other potential factors in a decision? Should what local competitors are doing enter into the discussion? How about the upcoming conference call with stock analysts? The relevancy condition requires that organizations focus on an explicit consideration of the values that should play a role in any decision. Involving wide groups of stakeholders in this process is critical for organizations, both for the role stakeholders play in blessing the decision framework suggested by the organization, and also because stakeholders will often introduce new perspectives that the organization would not have thought of on its own, perspectives that, when presented, are agreed upon as relevant to the discussion.

The third condition of accountability for reasonableness holds that decisions must be revisable in light of better rationales, including those generated by appeals procedures. More generally, a strong appeals structure must fit within an organized system for reflecting over time so that experience, better arguments, and further deliberation can lead to change. This structure for appeal, reflection, and revision overlaps with the tenets we introduced for organizational ethics and must be interwoven throughout all operational units of an exemplary health-care organization. Whether it is a medical necessity determination, a decision regarding the care of vulnerable populations, a strategic shift within community benefit programs, all must occur within an organizational culture and structure that *seeks* information through appeals and other measures and then *harnesses* that information for positive change.

Finally, the three substantive requirements for accountability for reasonableness—publicity, relevance, and revisability—must have some mechanism of enforcement. Both voluntary private enforcement and public agency regulation can help secure trust, in part through their watchdog functions, but also through facilitating broader public deliberation about the proper mechanisms for determining just limit-setting policies. In market-based health-care systems, public regulation has a distinctive additional role to play. Enforcing the features of procedural justice may leave wide disparities in the ways that organizations will prioritize competing ethical values. For instance, a for-profit health plan might take all the right steps to gain input, foster deliberation, and disclose rationales—and then announce it has decided to maximize its shareholder returns by minimizing its share of enrollees from poor sections of the community. Regulation is necessary to establish some basic minimums, some version of a level playing field, so that market competition does not lead to an ethical race to the bottom. Even if we were to assume that competitive markets eventually reward organizations that strike socially acceptable balances in producing value, health-care markets are notably imperfect; and if left unchecked, the lack of good information and of purchaser–consumer freedom may lead to competition that will strangle health-care organizations trying to do good and do well.

Taken in its entirety, then, the accountability-for-reasonableness framework connects health organization decisions to the broader educative and deliberative account of the democratic process (Gutmann and Thompson, 1996). If fulfilled consistently and robustly, the four conditions of accountability for reasonableness offer health-care organizations the chance to demonstrate that they exercise their authority to set priorities and limits in a legitimate fashion. They can partake of the legitimacy and trust of democracy itself.

In this book, our ethical analyses and interpretations of pragmatic examples from organizational experience have served to reinforce the importance and universal applicability of these tenets of procedural justice in health care. But our philosophical aim has been more audacious. We have sought to go beyond the procedural target of balancing ethical values toward the goal of elucidating central ethical obligations that should inform the solutions to problems of competing ethical values. Our lists of central ethical obligations set out landmarks for guiding organizations through the most critical choices to be made when confronting such problems. As normative statements, our lists of ethical obligations are vulnerable to the general philosophical skepticism that there can be any objective basis to moral judgments in a pluralistic society (Engelhardt, 1996). We argue, however, that the full deliberation inherent in the procedures required by accountability for reasonableness can actually lead the stakeholders in health-care organizations to a significant degree of moral consensus on key ethical obligations. The better the deliberation, the greater the chances of finding or building consensus. Our book has been an attempt, therefore, to link procedural justice in health care with its fruits: a growing awareness of the competing ethical values faced by health-care organizations; a deeper appreciation of the values and perspectives of others; a greater desire to work together to find solutions and learn from mistakes; and consequently, a stronger degree of consensus on guiding ethical principles and bedrock obligations.

THE "GOOD" HEALTH-CARE ORGANIZATION

Is there something missing still? Have we lost the forest for the trees? After considering the outlines of procedural justice and cataloguing every detail of examples that we could identify as exemplary, elucidating central ethical obligations to serve as bedrock principles while wrestling with competing ethical values, and laying out the structural requirements for ethical outcomes, have we yet captured the information necessary to help you decide whether you can trust your HMO?

We cannot conclude a discussion of organizational ethics without coming back to a perspective from which the history of ethics began: virtues. The accumulated virtues of an individual defines his or her character. For an organization, a sum of virtues is what constitutes its culture. Our experience examining the ethical structures and processes of many different health-care organizations left us with a profound respect for the day-to-day importance of organizational culture in determining the true trustworthiness of any organization. Hard to isolate, yet pervasive in its influence, organizational culture was the binding force that created an ethical whole out of an organization's many pieces.

We found that health-care organizations, even those in exactly the same line of business and in the same marketplace, often just *feel* very different on the inside. There really are distinctive and powerful mind-sets, ways of addressing people and problems, and visions of what makes for a good day at the office. A full discussion of the determinants and dynamics of organizational culture is outside the scope of this book, but our investigation led us to develop a strong normative sense of what characterizes the culture of the good health-care organization, and this normative picture lends substance and cohesion to our analysis of organizational ethics.

Guided, or biased perhaps, by our perspectives as clinicians, we propose that the good health-care organization recapitulates in its relationships—its relationships with purchasers, staff, clinicians, members, and the community—the best of the virtues found in the relationship between doctor and patient. Some organizations have a culture that exudes an intensity of connection, even a true affection, for its partners and its patients. Competent, respectful, honest, and kind; hearing equally the calls of compassion and those of justice; humble and desirous of learning from mistakes; attentive and accepting of accountability—all patients hope to find these qualities in their doctor. The outstanding health-care organization aspires to the same virtues in all its relationships.

This is our normative vision of a *caring organization*. The product of a caring organization is not shareholder value, nor risk management, nor even clinical services. Its product is caring relationships, and it bends its entire thought toward the achievement of that goal. It is the culture of the caring organization that acts like a pheromone, invisibly attracting and retaining like-minded caring individuals who find their own personal virtues affirmed time after time in their work experience. It is the culture that transmits organizational virtues into the toughest choices: the decisions over medical necessity, whether to care for vulnerable populations, and how much to invest in community benefit programs. With all the pieces of the ethical mosaic at its disposal, it is the culture of the caring organization that frames the larger picture.

And yet there are ways that specific exemplary ethical practices within an organization serve to build a positive organizational culture as well. The tools and approaches we have presented, especially those in the domains of consumer empowerment and organizational ethics, provide opportunities to exercise and strengthen the virtues of a caring organization. Listening, empowering, deliberating—just as in the individual, practicing these virtuous behaviors serves as its own reinforcement. In this way, the conceptions we have presented of procedural justice, central ethical obligations, and organizational culture form an integrated vision of the good health care organization.

LOOKING TOWARD THE FUTURE

In the setting of limited health-care resources, health-care organizations will face perennial ethical challenges. However, deliberating and deciding about how to manage competing ethical values cannot be left to even the most expert and benevolent clinicians and managers. Choosing priorities and setting health-care limits fairly requires clinical knowledge and managerial expertise, but the ultimate choices must inevitably reflect values choices as well as knowledge and expertise. These ethical choices must ultimately be made in accord with the values of the community.

In health-care systems that act in harmony with community values, the public will, over time, largely interpret limits as disappointing, but legitimate and fair. When systems function less well—as most observers believe is the case in the United States—stakeholders mistrust the limit-setting process and fight against it. The current U.S. trend towards shifting more of the financial risk in health insurance to enrollees reflects despair about the possibility of setting limits in a more collective manner that patients, providers, and the public can trust.

In the face of this apparent despair, the BEST project was inspired by a gleam of optimism. Perhaps, with so many natural experiments going on in the American health-care system, lessons could be learned that would enable health-care organizations and health systems to enhance the legitimacy of their policies and decisions. The BEST project was thus founded with a pragmatic perspective, looking to find how ethical theories and values fit with the landscape of the efforts and experience of different U.S. health-care organizations.

Did we find exemplary ethical practices, or did we manufacture exemplary practices out of the best that we could find? A pragmatic approach presupposes a dynamic moral environment: there will be no fixed end points with permanent ethical solutions, but rather a continuous process of engagement with changing circumstances. The exemplary ethical practices we have identified and characterized embody pragmatic, but virtuous, responses to the health-care environment in the United States in the late 1990s and the early years of this new century. A BEST project done in a different national context, or done 20 years from now in the United States, would show different pragmatic responses to different challenges.

We argue, however, that exemplary pragmatic responses to challenges of the future would embody the same core values that we developed as criteria for our analyses. The quest for ethical excellence in competitive markets will continue to find the values of individual care and those of population care in dynamic tension, a tension tempered always by the drive for sustainable profits. To meet this ethical tension, the centrality of procedural justice, the grounding function of central ethical obligations, and the role of organizational culture in determining ethical excellence will not change in 20—or 200—years.

Even philosophers adopting a pragmatic approach hope to uncover archetypal problems, find universal lessons, and achieve a lasting impact. The aim of this book has been to describe distinctive real-world approaches to perennial ethical challenges. We learned that the natural laboratories of American managed care do contain lessons for all health-care organizations and systems seeking ethical excellence in managing limited resources. We have provided health-care organizations, policy makers, consumers, and others alternative road maps to enhancing ethical performance. We hope most, however, to have contributed to a public dialogue about organizations and health care, a dialogue that must grow and deepen if it is ever to aspire to being a true deliberation. We are optimistic. Yet, there is much work to be done.

References

Academy for Health Services Research and Health Policy. (2001). *Choice: The "Hot Button" in Health Care?* Washington, DC: Academy for Health Services Research and Health Policy.

Acker. C. (1990). Treading Lighter on Byberry Closing. *Philadelphia Inquirer*, February 11, 1990, E1.

Aetna U.S. Healthcare. (1999). *Aetna's Brochure for Employers*. Available at http://www.aetnaushc.com/data/quality_managed_care99.pdf. Accessed June 5, 2000.

Anderlik, M. R. (2001). *The Ethics of Managed Care: A Pragmatic Approach*. Bloomington: University of Indiana Press.

Anders, G. (1996). *Health Against Wealth*. Boston: Houghton Mifflin.

Annas, G. J. (1998). *Some Choice: Law, Medicine, and the Market*. New York: Oxford University Press.

Attorney General, Commonwealth of Massachusetts. (2000). *The Attorney General's Community Benefits Guidelines for Health Maintenance Organizations*. Boston: Attorney General.

Baker, R. (2001). Bioethics and human rights: A historical perspective. *Cambridge Quarterly of Healthcare Ethics* 10:241–52.

Bergthold, L. A. (1995). Medical necessity: Do we need it? *Health Affairs* 4(4):180.

Biblo, J. D., Christopher, M. J., Johnson, L., and Potter, R. L. (1996). Ethical issues in managed care: Guidelines for clinicians and recommendations to accrediting organizations. *Bioethics Forum* 12(1):MC1–MC24.

Blake, D. C. (2000). Reinventing the healthcare ethics committee. *HEC Forum* 12:8–32.

Blendon, R., Leitman, I., Morrison, K., and Donelan, K. (1990). Satisfaction with health systems in ten nations. *Health Affairs* 9:185–92.

Brubaker, B. (2000). Sensitive Kaiser e-mails go astray. *Washington Post*, August 10, 2000, E1.

Bullen, B. (1998). *What Is a Prudent Purchaser?* Washington, DC: National Association of State Medicaid Directors.

Chassin, M., Kosecoff, J., Park, R. E., Winslow, C., Kahn, K., Merrick, N., Keesey, J., Fink, A., Solomon, D., and Brook, R. (1987). Does inappropriate use explain geographic variations in the use of health care services? A study of three procedures. *Journal of the American Medical Association* 258(18):2533–7.

Collins, J. C., and Porras, J. I. (1994). *Built to Last*. New York: Harper-Collins Publishers.

Collins, J. C., and Porras, J. I. (1996). Building your company's vision. In *Business Classics*. Boston: Harvard Business Review.

Daniels, N., and Sabin, J. E. (1997). Limits to health care: Fair procedures, democratic deliberation, and the legitimacy problem for insurers. *Philosophy and Public Affairs* 26(4):303–50.

Daniels, N., and Sabin, J. (2002). *Setting Limits Fairly*. New York: Oxford University Press.

Drucker, P. F. (1973). *Management: Tasks, responsibilities, practices*. New York: Harper and Row.

Dubinsky, J. E. (1997). What lawyers should know about business ethics. *Law Governance Review*, (summer). 13–23.

Eddy, D. M. (1996). Benefit language: Criteria that will improve quality while reducing costs. *Journal of the American Medical Association* 275(8):650–7.

Edgman-Levitan, S., and Cleary, P. D. (1996). What information do consumers want and need? *Health Affairs* 15(4):42–56.

Emanuel E. J. (1991). *The Ends of Human Life: Medical Ethics in a Liberal Polity*. Cambridge: Harvard University Press.

Emanuel, E. J., and Emanuel, L. L. (1992). Four models of the physician–patient relationship. *Journal of the American Medical Association* 267(16):2221–6.

Engelhardt, H. T. (1996). *The Foundations of Bioethics*, 2nd ed. New York: Oxford University Press.

Epstein, R. A. (1998). *Principles for a Free Society: Reconciling Individual Liberty with the Common Good*. Reading, MA: Perseus Books.

Ethical Force Program. (2000). *Protecting Identifiable Health Care Information Privacy: A Consensus Report on Eight Content Areas for Performance Measure Development*. Chicago: American Medical Association.

Faden, R. R., and Beauchamp, T. L. (1986). *A History and Theory of Informed Consent*. New York: Oxford University Press.

Fins, J. J., Miller, F. G., and Bacchetta, M. D. (1998). Clinical pragmatism: Bridging theory and practice. *Kennedy Institute of Ethics Journal* 8(1):37–42.

Forrow, L., Arnold, R. M., and Parker, L. S. (1993). Preventive ethics: Expanding the horizons of clinical ethics. *Journal of Clinical Ethics* 4:287–94.

Friedman, M. (1962). *Capitalism and Freedom*. Chicago: University of Chicago Press.

Fuchs, V. R. (1998). *Who Shall Live? Health, Economics, and Social Choice*. River Edge, NJ: World Scientific Publishing Co., Inc.

Goldsmith, J. (2000). The internet and managed care: A new wave of innovation. *Health Affairs* 19(6):42–56.

Goldstein, A., and Eilperin, J. (1998). House votes to increase rights of HMO patients; GOP leaders lose battle on lawsuits. *Washington Post*, October 8, 1998, A1.

Gostin, L. (1998). Health services research: Public benefits, personal privacy, and proprietary interests. *Annals of Internal Medicine* 129:833–5.

Grunwald, M. (1999). GOP doctors in the House put patients before party; Push for "Bill of Rights" irks leadership. *Washington Post*, July 27, 1999, A1.

Gutmann, A., and Thompson, D. (1996). *Democracy and Disagreement.* Cambridge: Harvard University Press.

Gutmann, A., and Thompson, D. (1997). Deliberating about bioethics. *Hastings Center Report* 27(3):38–41.

Hall, M., and Anderson, G. (1992). *Health Insurers' Assessment of Medical Necessity.* Philadelphia: University of Pennsylvania Law School.

Hasan, M. (1996). Let's end the nonprofit charade. *New England Journal of Medicine* 334(16):1055–7.

Health Net (2000). *Guide to Evidence-Based Medicine.* Available from Health Net, Medical Policy Communications Department, 3400 Data Drive, Rancho Cordova, CA 95670.

Health Privacy Project. Institute for Health Care Research and Policy. (1999). *Best Principles for Health Privacy: A Report of the Health Privacy Working Group.* Washington, DC: Georgetown University.

Hirschman, A. O. (1970). *Exit, Voice, and Loyalty: Responses to Decline in Firms, Organizations, and States.* Cambridge, MA: Harvard University Press.

Joint Commission for Accreditation of Healthcare Organizations. (2002). *Hospital Accreditation Standards.*

Kaiser Family Foundation. "Is There a Managed Care 'Backlash?'" November 5, 1997. Available at http://www.kff.org/content/archive/1328/mcarepr.num. Accessed May 23, 2000.

Kaiser Family Foundation. (1998). *External Review of Health Plan Decisions.* Report No. 1443. Prepared by Pollitz, K., Dallek, G., and Tapay, N. Washington, DC.

Kaiser Family Foundation. (2000). *External Review of Health Plan Decisions: An Update.* Report No. 3020. Prepared by Dallek, G., and Pollitz, K. Washington, DC.

Kaiser Family Foundation. (2002). *Assessing State External Review Programs and the Effects of Pending Federal Patients' Rights Legislation.* Report No. 3221. Prepared by Pollitz, K., Crowley, J., Lucia, K., and Bangit, E. Washington, DC.

Kassirer, J. P. (1995). Managed care and the morality of the marketplace. *New England Journal of Medicine* 333(1): 50–2.

Klein, S. A. (2000). AMA, TMA criticize Texas' legal settlement with Aetna. *American Medical News*, June 19, 2000, 5–6.

Master, R. J. (1998). Massachusetts Medicaid and the Community Medical Alliance: A new approach to contracting and care delivery for Medicaid-eligible populations with AIDS and severe physical disability. *The American Journal of Managed Care*, June 25, 4 Suppl:SP90–8.

McCarthy, E. (1999). Patients voice growing concern about privacy. *Sacramento Business Journal*, April 5, 1999, 26, 29.

McGee, G., ed. (1999). *Pragmatic Bioethics.* Nashville, TN: Vanderbilt University Press.

Mills, A. E., and Spencer, E. M. (2001). Organization ethics or compliance: Which will articulate values for the U.S. healthcare system? *HEC Forum* 13:329–43.

Monane, M., Mathias, D., Nagle, B., and Kelly, M. (1998). Improving prescribing patterns for the elderly through an online drug utilization review intervention: A system linking the physician, pharmacist, and computer. *Journal of the American Medical Association* 280(14):1249–52.

Moreno, J. D. (1995). *Deciding Together: Bioethics and Moral Consensus*. New York: Oxford University Press.

Morone, J. A. S., and Marmor, T. R. (1983). Representing consumer interests: The case of American health planning. In Marmor, T. R., *Political Analysis and American Medical Care*. Cambridge, UK: Cambridge University Press.

National Committee for Quality Assurance (NCQA). (2001). State of Managed Care Quality Report: 2001. Washington, DC. Available at http://www.ncqa.org. Accessed October 4, 2001.

Nudelman, P. M., and Andrews, L. M. (1996). The "value added" of not-for-profit health plans. *New England Journal of Medicine* 334(16):1057–9.

Ozar, D., Berg, J., Werhane, P. H., and Emanuel, L. (2000). *Organizational Ethics in Health Care: Toward a Model for Ethical Decision Making by Provider Organizations*. Chicago: American Medical Association Institute for Ethics.

Pear, R. (1997). Name-Calling Becomes Part of the Struggle to Define the Health Care Debate. *The New York Times*, 8 July 1997, A12.

Pritts, J., Goldman, J., Hudson, Z., Berenson, A., and Hadley, E. (1999). *The State of Health Privacy: An Uneven Terrain (A Comprehensive Survey of State Health Privacy Statutes)*. Health Privacy Project, Institute for Health Care Research and Policy. Washington, DC: Georgetown University.

Rawls, J. (1971). *A Theory of Justice*. Cambridge, MA: Harvard University Press.

Relman, A. S. (1992). What market values are doing to medicine. *Atlantic*. March, 98–102, 105–6.

Robinson, J. C. (2001). The end of managed care. *Journal of the American Medical Association* 285(20):2622–82.

Rodwin, M. A. (1997). The neglected remedy: Strengthening consumer voice in managed care. *American Prospect* 34:45–50.

Rosenbaum, S., Frankford, D. M., Moore, B., and Borzi, P. (1999). Who should determine when health care is medically necessary? *New England Journal of Medicine* 340(3):229–31.

Sabin, J. E., and Daniels, N. (1998). Making insurance coverage for new technologies reasonable and accountable. *Journal of the American Medical Association* 279(9): 703–4.

Sabin, J. E., and Daniels, N. (1999). Public sector managed behavioral health care: III. Meaningful consumer and family participation. *Psychiatric Services* 50:883–5.

Sabin, J. E., and Daniels, N. (2002). Strengthening the consumer voice in managed care: III. The Philadelphia Consumer Satisfaction Team. *Psychiatric Services* 53:23–24, 29.

Sabin, J. E., O'Brien, M. F., and Daniels, N. (2001). Strengthening the consumer voice in managed care: II. Moving NCQA standards from rights to empowerment. *Psychiatric Services* 52:1303–5.

Schlesinger, M., and Gray, B. (1998). A broader vision for managed care, Part 1: Measuring the benefit to communities. *Health Affairs* 17(3):152–68.

Schlesinger, M., Gray, B., Carrino, G., Duncan, M., Gusmano, M., Antonelli, V., and Stuber, J. (1998). A broader vision for managed care, Part 2: A typology of community benefits. *Health Affairs* 17(5):26–49.

Segal, D., and Goldstein, A. (1999). Tobacco lawyers aim at HMOs; Slew of suits expected to test law protecting managed care. *Washington Post*, October 1, 1999, E1.

Terry, K. (2000). What's in the box: Is UnitedHealthcare delivering on its promises? *Medical Economics*, September 4, 2000:158–71.

Wennberg, J. E., and Gittelsohn, A. (1973). Small area variations in health care delivery. *Science* 182(117):1102–8.

Wildt, A. (1999). Solidarity: its history and contemporary definition. In Bayertz, K., *Solidarity*, Dordrecht: Kluwer.

Wolf, S. M. (1994). Shifting paradigms in bioethics and health law: The rise of new pragmatism. *American Journal of Law & Medicine* 20(4):395–415.

Index